GLOBAL HEALING

THINKING OUTSIDE THE BOX

GLOBAL HEALING Trilogy by
VIPIN MEHTA

Book 1:

GLOBAL HEALING

Thinking Outside the Box

Book 2:

GLOBAL HEALING

Awakening Spirituality

Book 3:

GLOBAL HEALING

New Vistas of Hope

GLOBAL HEALING

THINKING OUTSIDE THE BOX

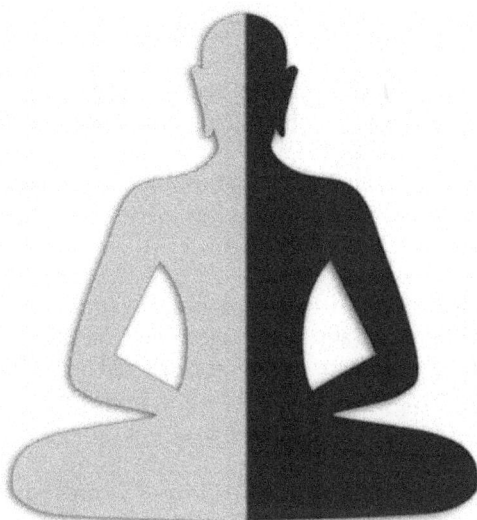

VIPIN MEHTA

Foreword by Harriet Fulbright

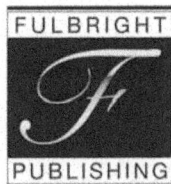

FULBRIGHT
F
PUBLISHING

Published by Fulbright Publishing, Inc., New York, New York

Design and Production by Helios Entertainment, New York, New York
www.heliosentertainment.com

Edited by Harriet Mayor Fulbright & Ravé Mehta

Photo courtesies from National Nuclear Security Administration/Nevada Site
Office; Time Magazine; other sources available upon request.

All diagrams in book are conceived by and remain the property of Vipin Mehta.
Special thanks to Radha Mehta, Andrea Russell and Alec Anderson for their
support.

Printed in the United States of America

Library of Congress Cataloging-in-Publication Data is available upon request

ISBN-13: 978-0-9755123-4-0

First Edition: 2007

CONTENTS

This book is dedicated to my Spiritual Friends who I call "Modern Mystics". I won't write their names, but they know to whom I refer. They are a fountain of inspiration. Their Love is Inexhaustible, Unbelievable and Unfathomable.

— *Vipin Mehta*

TABLE OF PICTURES AND FIGURES

ACKNOWLEDGEMENTS

In this lifetime, there are many who have supported me on my sacred journey towards Home, and although I will not be able to recognize everyone in a few short pages, I would like to send a blanket of gratitude to all who have participated and shared in my personal quest and the creation of this *Global Healing* book series.

I would like to thank my parents Chhotalal and Premkuvar Mehta for giving me LIFE in India during the period of the Independence Movement led by Mahatma Gandhi. During this period, spirituality had culminated throughout India. I was fortunate to be raised through adolescence under the influence of Mahatma Gandhi's experiments on truth and goodness to humanity. The truth he taught is that we, the members of the Global Family, are the children of Divinity, and we must treat each other respectfully, with love and care, by breaking the barriers of caste, color, ethnicity, and religious beliefs. Gandhi's life served as a role model from whom I learned lessons of courage, perseverance, and commitment.

I thank my Spiritual Master, J. Krishnamurthy, who introduced me to Metaphysics as a pathway to spirituality. He exposed me to the idea of transforming the Metaphysical matrix of emotional energy from negative to positive when I was 24.

I thank the incredible Mystic Poet Rabindranath Tagore, whose works I had imbibed since the age of 25. His writings opened my sense of beauty to experience Divinity. My fiancé then, now wife of over 37 years, joined me on this spiritual quest since this age and always stood by me year after year.

I thank the Mystic Rajneesh, globally known as Osho, who inspired me to be a seeker, at the age of 27, and to think and feel beyond the conformities of religious and spiritual scriptures.

I would like to specially and profoundly thank the Modern Mystics for giving me boundless, inexhaustible, and unfathomable love; for providing me a fountain of inspiration to write this book; and for teaching me how to consciously create my own reality. I sincerely thank Jach for giving himself so that the Modern Mystics can communicate with us. His contribution to humanity is enormous and truly amazing. I thank the staff of Concept Synergy for organizing and arranging seminars, workshops, and intensives in order for the Modern Mystics to share their knowledge with us. I have been attending these seminars for more than sixteen years while continuing to enrich my life by gaining knowledge of Metaphysics and spirituality. I have used my own interpretations and applications of this knowledge in writing this book, and I am responsible for that.

I thank my son Ravé for inspiring and persistently encouraging me to write this book. After the traumatic events of 9/11, I wanted to share my Metaphysical knowledge with humanity to awaken spirituality. It was my son who instilled in me the belief that I can share this knowledge and do so with courage. Ravé also introduced me to Mrs. Harriet Fulbright, a champion of humanitarian causes.

Harriet and I share an understanding of Metaphysics and have become spiritual friends while writing this book together. It was a long journey, and I sincerely appreciate her patience and ongoing encouragement while writing, reviewing, and editing this book.

I thank my daughter Radha, who is my hope in carrying the torch of spirituality to future generations. She has always brought laughter into my life with her smile, and has helped me continue this spiritual journey towards Home always with love, joy, and fun.

I thank Andrea Russell for her patience during the past five years in helping me organize and conduct research applicable to this book. I appreciate her talent of being able to understand what I saw in my imagination and for putting it into diagrams and figures. This book is my journey of perseverance and she always stood by me and kept me going.

Finally, I would like to thank my wife Hansa, who has been my fellow traveler on this sacred journey toward Home. She has constantly encouraged and supported me on all my spiritual endeavors, including this one. Without her support, I would not be the man I am today. There is truth that behind every successful man stands a powerful woman, which is surely my loving wife Hansa.

FOREWORD

by Harriet Mayor Fulbright

Vipin Mehta has written a book – a large book that became three – from his heart. Over the last several years, he has looked with growing dismay at the rise of animosity throughout societies, from local neighborhoods to countries to around the globe, and he feared for the very existence of civilization, as we know it. After months of intense thought and meditation, he began to develop an alternative to our march toward hostility and self-destruction and to write about the possibility of global healing from a spiritual and attitudinal viewpoint.

His ideas are deliberately inclusive; they lie outside the particulars of distinct religions or political structures. They can be understood and accepted by all religions, all political parties and ideologies, and by all races, tribes and citizens in all parts of this planet. They focus on the human ability to reach out to those who are different in upbringing, outlook, skin color and cultural orientation and to understand and accept those differences without feelings of threat or the need for combat.

There should be no surprise in the making of a connection between the ideas of Senator J. William Fulbright and Vipin Mehta. Although the vocabularies used by the two men are different, Fulbright's focus on politics – government and the law and international diplomacy and Mehta's thesis based on the human mind and spirituality are in concert and moves us toward the same end-state – a more peaceful and integrated global community.

Fulbright began to focus on peaceful dialogue early on in his career and gained nationwide recognition for initiating the resolution that led to the establishment of the United Nations, which helped him win a place in the

US Senate representing the state of Arkansas in 1944. His aim was to create an international organization that would encourage nations to discuss their differences before they heated up to the boiling point and led to irreparable hostilities.

Two years later, toward the end of World War II, the United States dropped atomic bombs on Japan, and it was clear that this new weapon brought warfare to a far more destructive level than ever before in history. To study the long-term effects of the event, Fulbright called to the Senate chambers not only military and political experts to testify but physicians, psychologists, environmentalists and the scientists who created the bomb. What he heard so appalled him that he felt compelled to look for some means, any means, of preventing another world war. Atomic warfare was no longer an acceptable continuation of politics by other means. He firmly believed that in a world with nuclear weapons, the enemy cannot be destroyed because the true enemy is war itself.

The program which grew out of the hearings is the one he considered his greatest accomplishment: namely, the international education exchange program that bears his name, signed into law by President Truman on August 1, 1946. It became clear to him, especially as he looked back on his experiences as a Rhodes Scholar, that if future leaders from every country could come to know one another and learn to exchange ideas, then perhaps they might not be so willing to exchange bullets.

In the third and final book in the *Global Healing* series, "*Global Healing – New Vistas of Hope*", Vipin Mehta has made an invaluable contribution to the struggle toward a global plan for the achievement of a peaceful society focused on constructive collaborative activity. His ideas mesh perfectly with Senator Fulbright's ideas and the international education exchange program that bears his name, for as he said in his last book, *The Price of Empire*,

"The great strength and enduring value of the Fulbright program has been its ability to work patiently and persistently to build human networks around the globe."

These networks are essential because the path toward a peaceful world must be paved by those with the ability to listen, to understand differing ways of thinking, and to change minds through persistent persuasion rather than by force. As Fulbright said,

"In our quest for world peace the alteration of attitudes is no less important, perhaps more important, than the resolution of issues. It is in the minds of men, after all, that wars are spawned; to act upon the human mind, regardless of the issue or occasion for doing so, is to act upon the source of conflict and the potential source of redemption and reconciliation.

Extreme nationalism and dogmatic ideology are luxuries that the human race can no longer afford. It must turn its energies now to the politics of survival. If we do so, we may find in time that we can do better than just survive. We may find that the simple human preference for life and peace has an inspirational force of its own, less intoxicating perhaps than the sacred abstractions of nation and ideology, but far more relevant to the requirements of human life and human happiness."

As you will see when you read this book, Vipin Mehta points us toward what he calls the *New Age of Dominion* – in other words, toward the same setting for happiness and the chance for fulfillment that Senator Fulbright spent his life pursuing.

Chapter 1

INVITATION

Humanity is at a crossroad. At this point in our history we face two paths - two possibilities. It is a simple choice. Either we choose to commit Global Suicide by continuing to fight each other with ever more powerful and poisonous weapons, or we can turn toward a path of Global Healing. Years ago a famous scientist issued a warning:

> *"I can't tell you how the 3rd world war will be fought, though I can tell you how the 4th will be...with sticks and stones."*
> *- Albert Einstein*

Einstein was right: if we embark on a 3rd World War with nuclear weapons and other weapons of mass destruction, then we make the choice of committing Global Suicide and destroying civilization as we know it. Some people may think that this is an inevitable calamity, but it is not.

We would be choosing it. If we have the ability to choose Global Suicide then we also have the ability to choose the path of Global Healing.

Now is the time for revolution ---
Revolution of thinking outside the box with a new kind of knowledge.
Revolution of feeling outside the box by using new senses
listening to the inner voice, the soul's voice.

The soul has been crying for the last 60 years
each time there was violence, injustice, discrimination and misery.
The soul has been sending messages to humanity
through whispers and inner voices.
Now, the soul of humanity, which has been wounded,
sends us messages through screams and shouts.
It is telling us that the dark cloud of global suicide is ready
to envelope and crush us.
Now is the time to implement new knowledge and approaches,
with a deeper sense of love and caring for global healing.

Welcome to all our friends and fellow human beings on this journey to explore a new approach for Global Healing while creating a new man, a peaceful man, a loving and caring man that will lead us toward a new and evolved civilization. We must open our inner senses and explore feeling "outside the box" that constrains our current thinking. We must learn to listen to our inner voices, our soul's voices which gives us messages in various ways - over the whispers, screams and shouts from those bent on Domination and leading us toward Global Suicide. If we, humanity at large, do not act now, and take responsibility for our future, the forces for war and Domination will prevail.

We create our own Reality
and we are Responsible for what we are
at this crossroad of global suicide versus global healing.

United we stand ---
United, all of us unique and diverse, stand for global healing.
All diversities are beautiful and musical
if all of us, in our own diverse ways, are in Harmony.

Divided we fall --
Divided, we of all persuasions, glide helplessly toward global suicide.

All conflicts are ugly and violent
if we are divided by arrogance and isolation leading to dissonance.

As human beings, whatever diverse communities we belong to, we are all stakeholders and participants. Whether you belong to any one of the myriads of political, ideological or religious groups, this is the time to turn from those perspectives and focus on saving humanity from our current self-destructive path.

- You may be rich or poor; white collar or blue collar;
- You may be white, black, red, yellow or brown;
- You may be American, Latin, European, African, Asian or Middle Eastern;
- You may be a scientist or man of cloth; a public official or a businessman;
- You may be male or female; heterosexual or gay;

Regardless of the category, we are all human and we share the same planet.

5

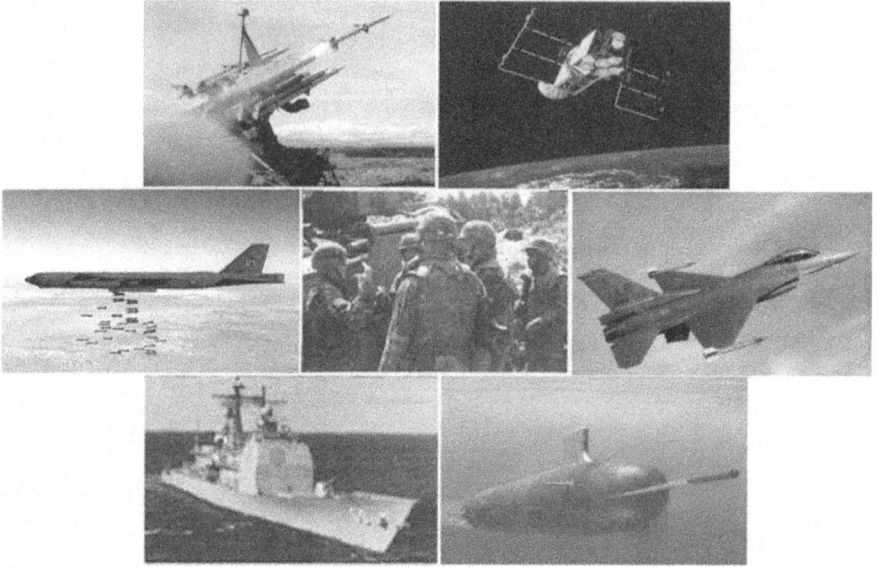

The worldwide military budget is over $1 trillion annually

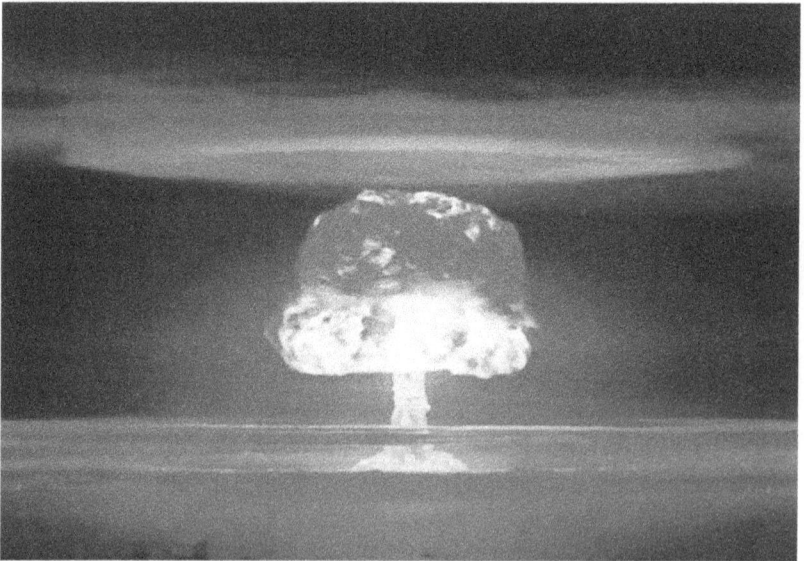

**The explosive power of the world's nuclear arsenal is equal to
one million Hiroshima bombs**

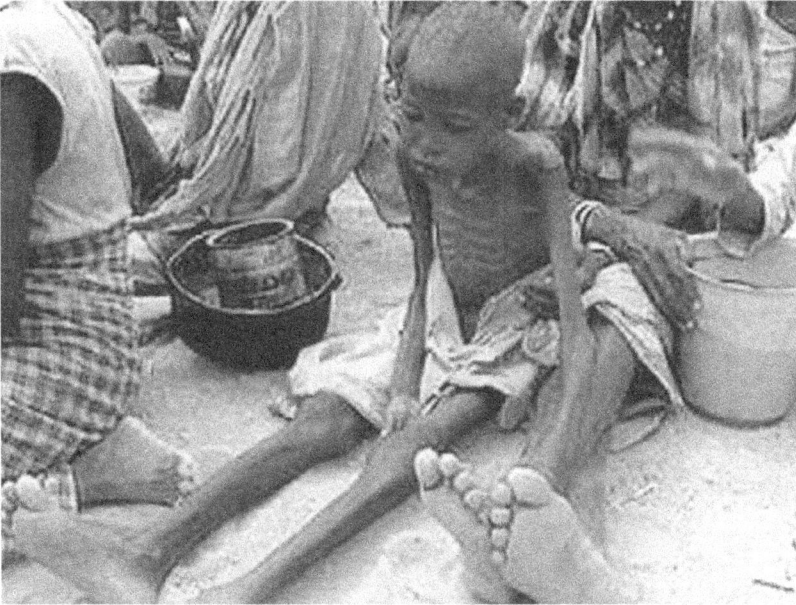

800 Million People (13% of mankind) suffers from dire hunger or malnutrition; 24,000 People die each day because of lack of food

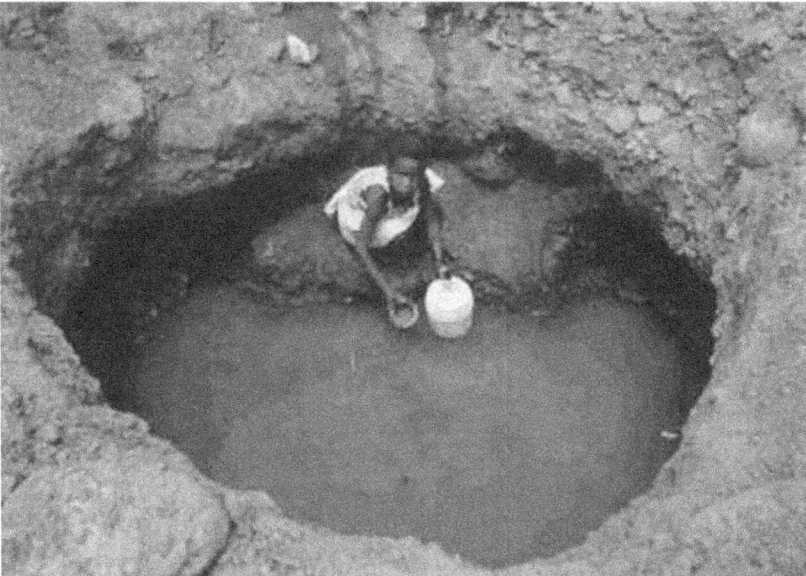

Over 1 billion people lack access to clean water and nearly 2 billion lack access to sanitation

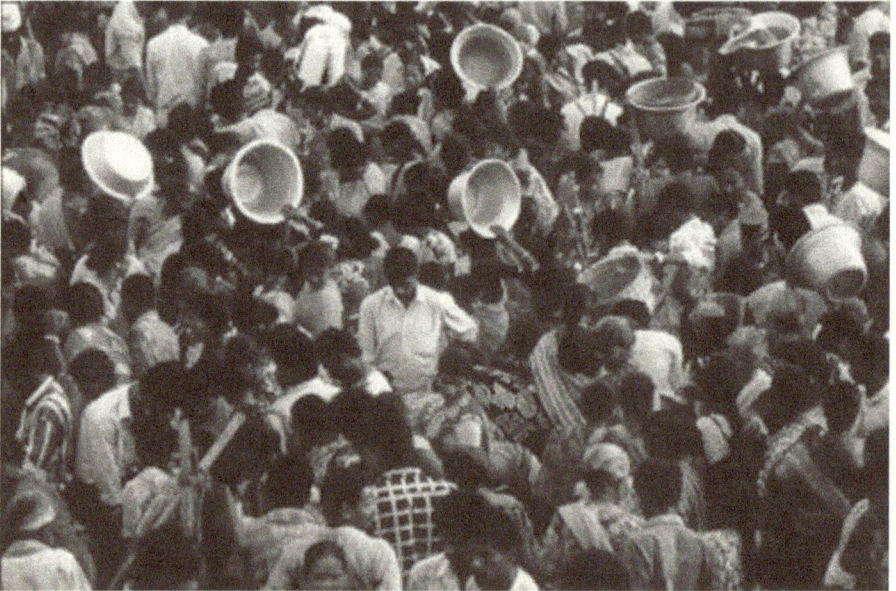

The world's population will increase by 728 million people over the next 10 years

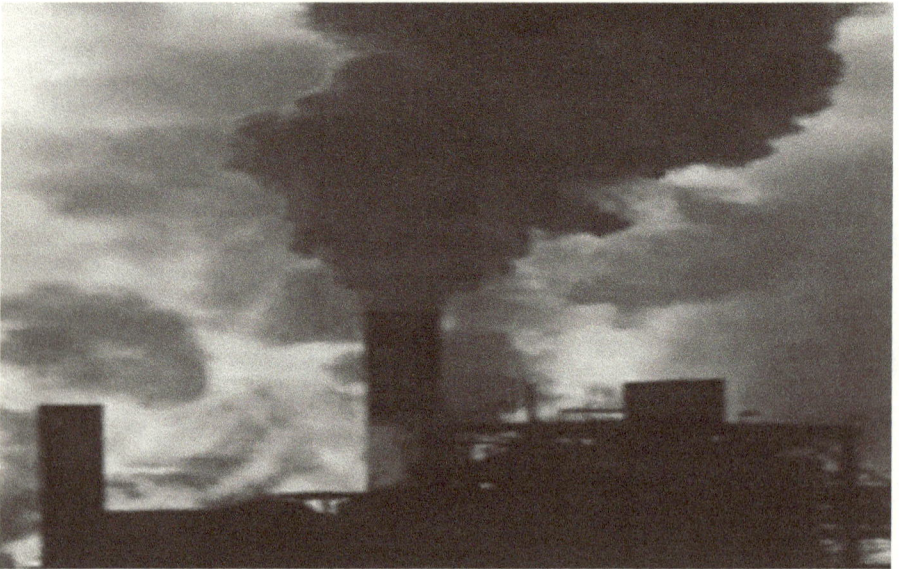

25% of the world's population consumes 75% of the world's primary energy

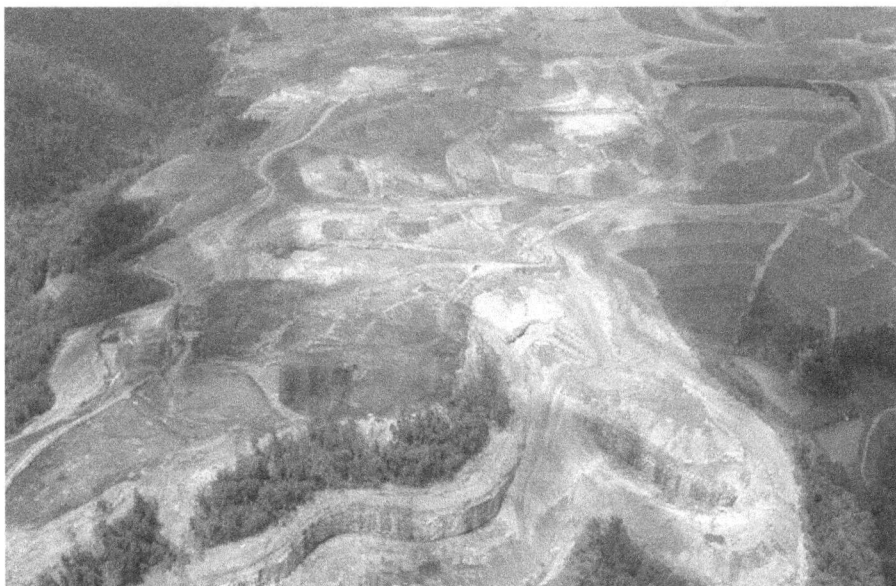

16.1 Million Hectares of forest are destroyed annually

What are we, humanity, doing?

The stock piling of weapons of mass destruction alone demonstrates that man is not yet civilized. Behind those weapons there are human minds. The minds that can appreciate the beauty of a rose and the splendor of love cannot hoard weapons that can cause massive deaths or destroy our planet.

Since we are all human beings, now is the time to set all the differences aside and take the pilgrimage of Global Healing.

> *The diversity of religious beliefs is as beautiful as a rainbow.*
> *We must respect each other's beliefs and learn from them.*
>
> *At the same time,*
> *The diversity of religious beliefs can become ugly and violent*
> *if those beliefs divide us and create isolation and arrogance*
> *when the convictions are:*
>
> *"Our belief system is purer than your belief system.*
> *Our God is holier than your God.*
> *Our God is the only God.*
> *Our religion is better than your religion.*
> *If we die for our religion we will go to heaven.*
> *This is our Jihad."*

Whether you believe in God or believe there is no God, now is the time for all of us to learn, respect and understand the intent of each other's religious beliefs for the common cause of humanity.

Mankind has never been at such a critical moment such as today. There have been thousands of battles and wars, but they did not destroy all life. Today, a few maniacal leaders amass weapons of mass destruction and can destroy the whole civilization. A nuclear war and war with weapons of mass destruction simply means total destruction, total devastation, a total man-made catastrophe. Nobody is going to be victorious; instead we are all preparing our own graves. Now is the time to assume responsibility by actively participating in the decision-making process. This is not only a matter of our evolution; it is a matter of our existence.

We can awaken the will and the means
to direct science and technology toward humanitarian aims.

We can develop the attitudes
which will transform human divisions
into harmonic diversity.

We can redirect human consciousness toward
changing the course of life
from global suicide to global healing.

The terrorist attack on September 11th was one of those cataclysmic once-in-a-generation life-changing events. The declaration of this war was without precedence. In the past, war has always been declared against a state or nation, and the rules of conduct were drawn up at the Geneva Convention. In this case, the "war" was initiated by a band of terrorists whose allegiance was not to a state, but to an ideal, and their "home" was not rooted in a physical territory, but in a belief.

This is a journey humanity must take because of the terrorist acts which have increased in number and intensity over the last half-century. We must strive to understand what motivates the perpetrators of such acts and why the traditional violent response to terrorism simply inspires further violence. We must think "outside the box" to bring an end to a hatred so extreme that a human is compelled to kill innocent women and children and even themselves. This journey requires courage, but promises great rewards.

Courage means going into the unknown
in spite of all fears.
Courageous people confront their fears and forge ahead.
Going into the unknown gives them a thrill.
Hearts start pulsing faster,
and every fiber of their being feels full of life
because they have accepted the challenge of the unknown.

Courage is risking the shift from the known to the unknown;
risking the passage from the familiar to the unfamiliar;
giving up the comfortable for the uncomfortable.
It is an arduous pilgrimage to an unknown destination.
In truth it is gambling,
and only gamblers really know the fullness of life.

Now is the time to be courageous;
to depart from the known, the familiar and the comfortable.
To turn away from the collective mind of
thinking that war and Domination over terrorists
are the only answers.

It is time to embrace the unknown, the unfamiliar and the
uncomfortable;
to embark on the pilgrimage toward "thinking outside the box"
to achieve global healing and to win the war on terrorism.

This type of journey is not entirely new to the human race. Columbus embarked on an arduous voyage over the uncharted waters of the ocean and found America. Mahatma Gandhi listened to the soul's voice and led India in a non-violent movement to gain freedom from the British for his people. Dr. Martin Luther King also listened to his inner voice. Through inspiring speeches and adherence to the law, he was able to begin the liberation of minorities from discrimination by forcing the passage of the Civil Rights Act through peaceful means. In South Africa Nelson Mandela also heard the call and suffered through 28 years of prison to free his people from the oppression of apartheid.

Humanity has come to this crossroad as a result of the limitations and boundaries set by ourselves. It is time to use persuasion and humanitarian aid instead of force, to listen with respect and caring rather than to deliver ultimatums, to turn toward methods of healing and lay down weaponry. Now is the time to use the power of choice to shift our path towards Global Healing.

Senator Fulbright once said, "In our quest for world peace the *alteration of attitudes* is no less important, perhaps more important, than the resolution of issues. It is in the minds of men, after all, that wars are spawned; to act upon the human mind, regardless of the issue or occasion for doing so, is to act upon the source of conflict and the potential source of redemption and reconciliation."

In essence, the *Global Healing* series is an exploration on how to change the human mindset, and in doing so change the world. To accomplish this we must first understand our current thinking process and then explore a deeper understanding of how the mind itself works.

Chapter 2

THINKING INSIDE THE BOX

We, humanity at large, approximately six billion people, have relinquished our responsibility for thinking and decision making to a handful of political, military, financial and religious leaders. By giving our power to leaders, we are told what to do by somebody else, and we abdicate all responsibility. These leaders are actively involved in making choices and decisions for us and selecting approaches for winning the war on terrorism and establishing global peace. The methods they use to implement their policies have been practiced for hundreds of years. Current leaders use politics, diplomacy, military might, economic pressure, and religion to set our course for the future. These leaders hold powerful positions because millions of people depend on them for guidance.

We need to bear in mind that some leaders also have their own vested interests in retaining power either personally or collectively. They care about their fame and historical importance. Each one has a personal agenda and a desire to control, rule and to exert power over others. These vested interests narrow their vision, which in turn creates conflicts and collisions within society at large, dividing humanity.

17

Historical Background

In the 20th century we have witnessed how science and technology has developed in leaps and bounds through exercising 'out of the box' thinking. Unfortunately, we have not paid adequate attention to the evolution of human relations. In fact, the development of human relations and human consciousness should be the highest priority where science and technology's primary role is to be the engine that drives humane progress, not lead it. Instead, science and technology has been thrown billions of dollars and as a result developed much faster than our ability to get along and understand each other. Without human consciousness at the helm steering the ship, we have navigated ourselves into a perfect storm where the Ark of Humanity will end in a global shipwreck unless we quickly and carefully veer ourselves into calmer waters! Let's explore some historical highlights to see how we arrived to our present state.

Human Invention:

In 1902, the Wright brothers made their miraculous flight of 120 feet, in a double winged plane capable of carrying only the pilot, and it started a revolution in transportation. Since that time many have flown faster than the speed of sound, across oceans and to all parts of the planet. Several have even made it to the moon and back. Even on the ground, within this century, people can now travel a mile a minute or faster on wheels instead of on foot or by animal, revolutionizing daily life everywhere.

Discoveries in the field of physics have been equally extraordinary and have transformed our understanding of man, matter and the universe. Shortly after the turn of the century, Einstein announced the development of his theory of relativity, which totally changed the way we look at the world. Scientists have since studied our planetary system and the universe beyond, using not only powerful telescopes but also space satellites with the capacity to travel millions of miles beyond our atmosphere. They have at the same time performed extraordinary studies on particles so small we can know them only by the trails they leave. This research has led to discoveries about a power source more magically beneficial and at the same time more destructive than anyone could have ever imagined a century ago.

And just a few years after the Wright brothers and Einstein made the news, the first national radio program was broadcast in the United States, marking the beginning of mass communication. High technology now delivers not only sound, but images worldwide; a news event is communicated via satellite within seconds of its happening to radios and television sets on every continent. Big governments and businesses are not alone in their ability to gather news and spread information. Millions of individuals can turn on their computers or pick up their telephones and interact with those they have never met face to face, to conduct research, join together in campaigns, or just enjoy conversations. To give you one example of the power this gives each individual, Jody Williams in the small New England town of Putney, Vermont, launched a worldwide campaign against land mines and, armed with only a phone, fax machine and a computer, succeeded in convincing the heads of 80 countries to sign a treaty banning their future use. She received the Nobel Peace Prize for her work.

Modern medicine is now close to making the bionic human a reality. Transplants of hearts, livers, kidneys and other vital organs are now commonplace, and miracle medicines are bringing people with life threatening diseases back from the brink of death. The cloning of animals is a reality, which means to many that the cloning of human beings is at least within the realm of possibility whether we like it or not.

Clearly those who have chosen to make science, mathematics, medicine or technology their life work had to abandon traditional ways of thought to make the big leaps and bounds. They have listened to the words of Robert Kennedy, have dreamed the impossible and have learned how to make it happen. They have released themselves from the constraints of thinking "inside the box."

Human Relations:

As we explore the journey of humanity during the 20th century, we can see that there were two main periods. One was preparation of war and the second was actual war itself.

The 20th century started with the preparation for war leading up to the first World War. That was the most destructive fighting up to that time, and it left Europe exhausted and destitute. A farsighted group of leaders proposed the formation of an international body called the League of Nations to prevent another world conflict, but the United States would not join, and the effort languished and finally collapsed. Again preparations for war began, and we entered into the second World War, which spread far wider and was more destructive than World War I, ending with the use of atomic bombs.

Then came the formation of the United Nations followed by the Cold War era. During this time, from the late 1940's to 1991, the world's major powers created arsenals of nuclear and conventional weapons. Each country developed powerful espionage organizations and engaged in limited confrontations and battles, including Korean War, India-China War, Cuban Missile Crisis, India-Pakistan War and Vietnam War. There were also limited attempts to settle differences: the formation of Bangladesh, USSR Missile Treaty, freedom of Poland, collapse of the Berlin Wall, the breakup of the USSR, and the struggle of Eastern Europe toward freedom and democracy.

Since 1950 there has been continual violence and cease-fires between

Israel and Palestine, and they have not arrived at any solution because of the current thinking and mindset of both sides. There has also been a continuous increase in terrorist activity. Another ongoing conflict has been between India and Pakistan over Kashmir issues with threats of terrorism, government action, and Nuclear Warfare.

It's time to sincerely ask the questions:

Where are we going?
What are our aims?
Nuclear war?
The third world war with weapons of mass destruction?
Global Suicide?

Humanity at large: Are we learning anything from history or just repeating old patterns with ever more powerful weapons and technology, working towards creating a bigger man-made cataclysm? It appears that humanity spent the 20th century, either preparing for war or fighting wars under the guise of establishing peace. All of the knowledge and methodologies, information, research and analysis, logic and reason, negotiation, treaties and cease-fires have not worked. On the contrary, all the erudition, knowledge and approaches have brought us to a worse possible outcome: Nuclear Warfare.

In less than 150 years we have gone from a global population of 1 billion souls to one that is about 6 billion, and more than 75% of the world's population live in underdeveloped countries where hunger and poverty are the norms.

Our ability to get along with each other and govern ourselves is also at a new low. The last century is noted for two of the most destructive world wars in recorded history and a desperate worldwide depression in between, followed by forty years of cold war, when two great powers spent billions of dollars on developing and manufacturing missiles which could end all life on the planet, not just once, but many times over. Even now, there are many hot battles in progress, often among people who have lived side by side as neighbors for generations.

This leads us to a fundamental paradox about human nature: as the world becomes more and more a global village, its inhabitants become less unified and more focused on "narrower identities".

Formation of the United Nations:
At the height of the Second World War, Senator J. William Fulbright, remembering that his country had quickly returned to its isolationist stance after World War I, drew up a resolution for the formation of an international body on the order of the failed League of Nations and persuaded the leaders of both parties in Congress to support it so that it passed both Houses by a landslide vote.

Shortly after the cessation of the hostilities, representatives from 50 countries met in San Francisco at a gathering called the United National Conference on International Organizations to draw up the United Nations Charter. The first proposals were worked out beforehand at Dumbarton Oaks in Washington, DC, by delegates from China, the Soviet Union, the United Kingdom, and the United States, from August to October in 1944. Less than one year later on June 26, 1945, the 50 representatives signed the United Nations Charter. Poland, which was not represented at the west coast conference, signed later and became one of the original 51 Member States.

The vision of an international body composed of all the major countries of the world, ready and able to improve collaboration among nations, deter hostilities between nations with conflicting agendas, was an exciting forward-looking initiative. Its purpose was to bring all nations of the world together based on the principles of justice, human dignity and the well being of all people. Its aims were:

> - To keep the peace throughout the world;
> - To develop friendly relations between nations;
> - To work together to help people live better, to eliminate poverty, disease and illiteracy in the world, to stop environmental destruction and to encourage respect for each other's rights and freedoms;
> - To be a center for helping nations achieve these goals.

The issue hampering the organization from the beginning was national sovereignty. Each country was only willing to cooperate as a supreme entity, not subject to the laws or court decision of the umbrella organization. Thus, the principles hammered out among the members were:

> - All members states have sovereign equality;
> - All member states must try to settle their differences by peaceful means;
> - Countries must avoid the use of force or threats to use force;
> - The UN may not interfere in the domestic affairs of any country;
> - All countries should try to assist the United Nations in their work.

When these principles were signed, it was acknowledged that none of the resolutions passed by the United Nations would be binding on any nations, but it was hoped that the weight of world opinion would be enough to keep each country in line. Unfortunately, human nature and age-old habits has kept the body from fully achieving its purpose. The prevalence of thinking "inside the box" has prevented many important resolutions from passing, and weakened many others that did pass, but were ignored or merely given lip service.

This is not to say that the United Nations has failed. Its work in the educational, social and cultural fields have been important, and the fact that there is an institution promoting dialogue between nations has been important as a neutral ground for airing issues. Nevertheless, it could serve the world more effectively with a strong world court, a permanent peacekeeping force, and a primary focus on promotion of those elements that improve human well-being.

The current conventional and traditional thinking, using traditional politics, diplomacy, negotiations, military might, economic pressure and religious concepts are all a long-held habit of thinking "inside the box", and has drawn humanity, with the passage of time, closer and closer to Global Suicide. Thinking "inside the box" has kept us from understanding what fundamentally stands in the way of peace and human progress. A focus on how to improve daily life for all requires breaking the confines of our present set of ideas and our current mode of doing the people's work.

So, fellow explorers, now is the time to cut the ties to traditional approaches, and take back our responsibility from our leaders and call upon our own courage to step into the unknown.

Courage is not only the opposite of cowardice; it is also breaking through the current conformity of thinking.

In general, people are more comfortable with consistency rather than change. It is easier to go through daily life following established patterns instead of inventing new methods, finding new paths, creating different structures, and dreaming up new ideas to accomplish tasks. We must call upon our imaginations, dream impossible dreams, and break the narrow boundaries of our traditional ways of thought. We need to seek the objectivity and observation of scientists, the hearts of poets, the visions of painters, the balance and harmony of musicians and the wisdom of philosophers. We have to expand beyond our current forms of knowledge and come up with innovative, inventive and imaginative approaches to turn humanity away from our current path.

Chapter 3

HIERARCHY OF KNOWLEDGE

What is "knowledge"? According to the Webster Dictionary, the definition of knowledge has a wide range of meanings such as: "a clear and certain perception of something; the act, fact, the state of knowing; understanding; learning - all that has been perceived or grasped by the mind; practical experience, skill; acquaintance or familiarity (with a fact or place); cognizance, recognition; information; the body of facts accumulated by mankind; acquaintance with facts; range of awareness or understanding."

Knowledge and understanding are essential for human co-existence with Mother Nature, which includes the mineral, plant and animal kingdoms. Compared to animals, our physical traits come up short. They see better, hear better, and their sense of smell is significantly more developed. They run faster and are stronger. They are well equipped to exist in extreme weather conditions such as hurricanes, storms, floods and a wide fluctuation of temperature changes. However, we, humans, are gifted with special inner faculties: the ability to think and feel a wide range of emotions; to perceive and to have perception; to conceive and have conception; to remember and record memories; to imagine and to have dreams and visions; to have passion and to become compassionate; and to love and to care. It is with these unique gifts that we can explore knowledge.

The human population consists of 6 billion people, and each individual is at a different stage in life acquiring different levels of knowledge. For simplified understanding of the many dimensions and directions of knowledge, knowledge is classified into five types (see figures *"Hierarchy of Human Knowledge" and "Bell Curve of Knowledge"*). The first three are products of the human mind: information, intellect and intelligence, and ESP (extra sensory perception). With the progress of science, technology and psychology in the 20th century, humanity has accepted that these exist.

The fourth type of knowledge is called Metaphysics. Fundamentally, the brain exists within the space-time dimension and is considered physical, however the mind exists beyond the space-time dimension and is therefore Metaphysical. Metaphysics is the knowledge of the human mind in its total complexity and understanding the body-mind-soul-spirit relationship in pursuit of betterment of oneself and humanity. Metaphysics is also the spiritual science of changing negative thoughts and feelings to positive, such as 'hate' to 'love'. Metaphysics is explored by people who seek spirituality, traditionally referred to as 'seekers' and in modern spirituality known as 'Metaphysicians'. In the pursuit of spirituality, the Metaphysician becomes a spiritual being and experiences a glimpse of enlightenment. In the 21st century, it is this type of knowledge that will guide human consciousness back to the forefront of science and technology and move humanity toward a path of Global Healing.

Hierarchy of Human Knowledge

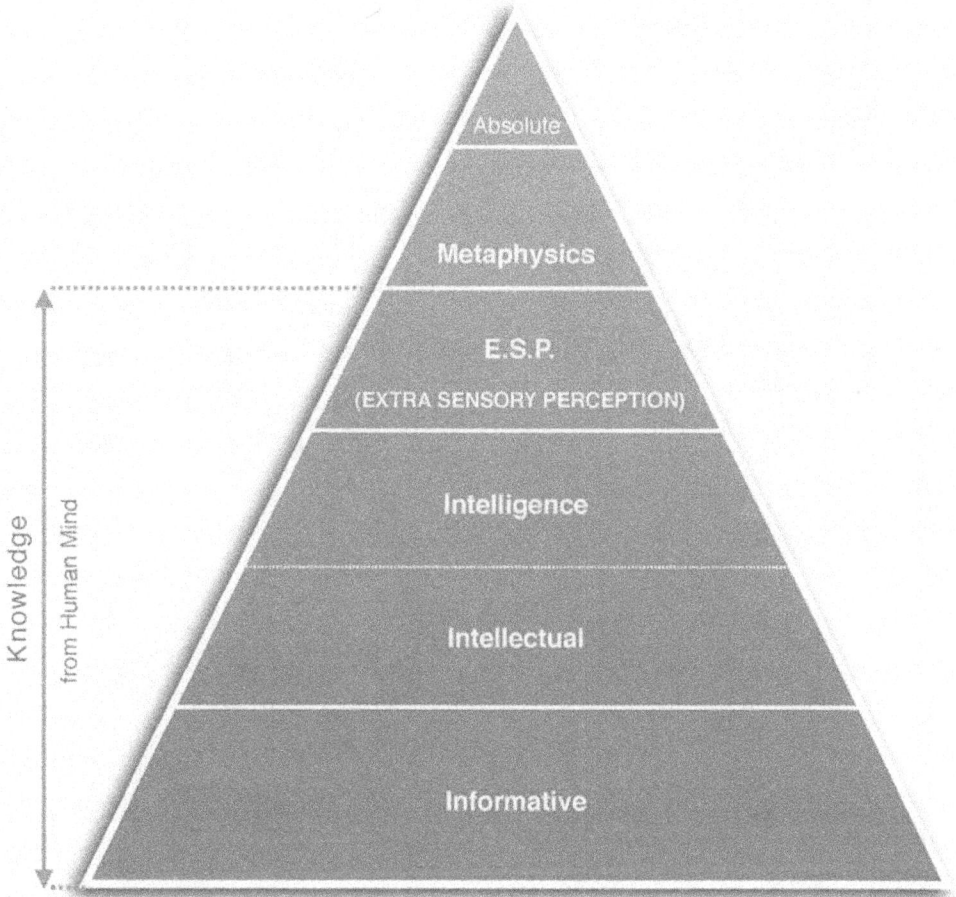

Bell Curve of Knowledge

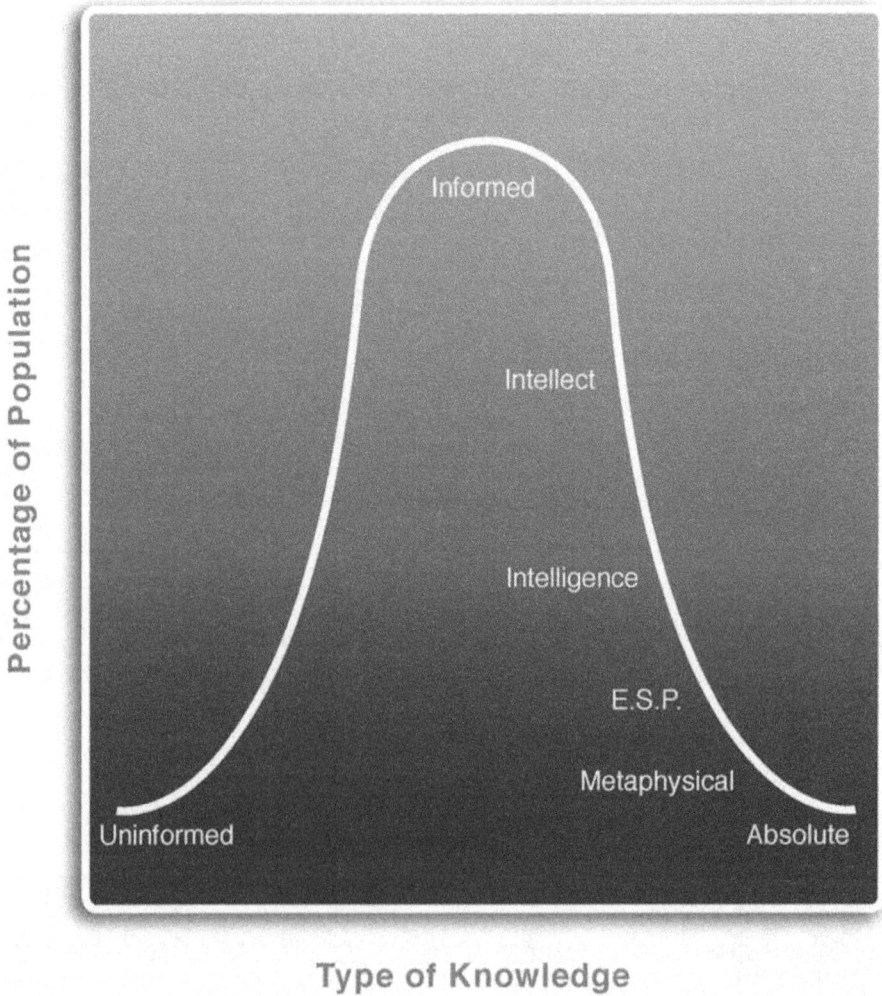

Percentage of Population

Informed

Intellect

Intelligence

E.S.P.

Metaphysical

Uninformed

Absolute

Type of Knowledge

The fifth type of knowledge is absolute knowledge, which is attained by enlightened masters often referred to as messiahs, prophets or bhagwans as well as other names.

Let us explore these five types of knowledge in more detail.

Information

We are familiar with information, the first type of knowledge, because we have been living in the information age for the last century. The dictionary meaning of information is "to give form to, to represent, inform: an informing or being informed, of telling or being told of something; knowledge acquired in any manner: facts, data, learning, lore." The Metaphysical meaning of information is "energy in formation, thought energy or thought in formation".

Human beings have basically five familiar senses, sight/seeing, sound/hearing, smell, touch and taste. These senses are the doorways to life (see figure "*Internet of Human Senses – Doorways to Life – Part 1*"). From these five senses, human beings collect information and pass it on to the brain. According to modern science, information collected by all senses except smell passes through the temporal lobe to the cerebral cortex, then to the right and left lobes. Smell is the only sense that goes directly to the cerebral cortex. The brain processes the information it receives and passes it to the mind. The mind reacts or responds to this information, makes choices and decisions according to the current mindset, and then acts upon the processed information.

Information or informative knowledge is received through many sources: people, radio, television, books, magazines, newspapers, movies, photographs, advertisements and other means of audio and visual communication. Informative knowledge is not authentic knowledge

Internet of Human Senses
Doorways to Life – Part 1

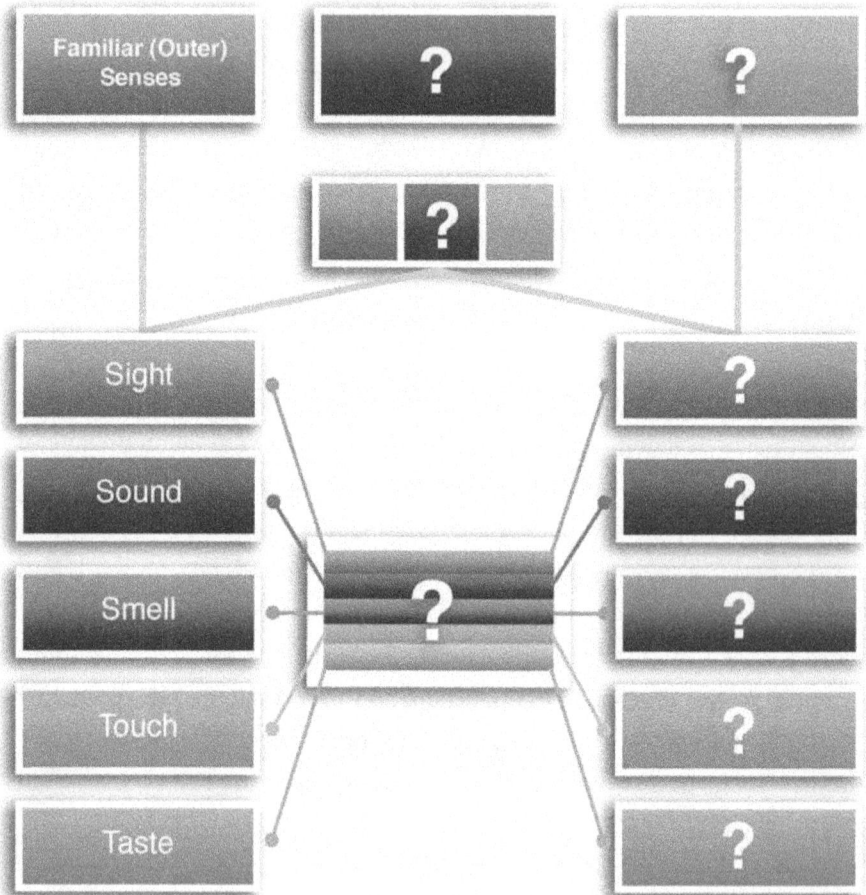

because it is not experienced first hand at the heart or soul level. People who focus on informative knowledge tend to become teachers, professors, pundits, scholars and priests, but they never become "knowers" – those who have gained their knowledge through their own personal experience.

The majority of knowledge imparted in the traditional education system is informative knowledge. This knowledge becomes a part of memory. It is like a recording or video played again and again. For instance, if "God exists" or "there is no God" is told again and again, then the memory becomes stronger and stronger until at some point people start believing it. They forget that it has been recited to them and it is not a first hand experience. However, informative knowledge, the lowest level in the knowledge hierarchy, is important because it sets the foundation for mass psychology.

In the 20th century there was a great explosion of information. The speed of creating and passing information was accelerated from letter delivery by horseback, to the telegraph, telephone, fax, email, audio/video conferencing and from a physical library of books to the internet. This communication has brought people together, illustrated by the real-time worldwide celebration of the millennium from the sunrise of Japan to the sunset of Hawaii. In this information age revolution, the poor and rich have equal access to information through all forms of communication.

This has created a major shift in the political, economical, social, scientific and religious power structures. Politically, individuals now have more opportunities to share and express their opinions about major decisions, such as the war in Iraq. Economically, information has become a more valuable commodity than even natural resources as seen on Wall Street. Socially, people have been exposed to more choices in connecting and establishing relationships despite national, ethnic, racial or religious boundaries. Science and technology have mushroomed because information is instantly available. With regard to religion, people have easier access to explore different scriptures, beliefs, religions and other information pertaining to spirituality.

This explosion of information has also come with curses. There have been abuses of informative knowledge in the form of distortions and exaggerations, scandals and inappropriate disclosures. In addition, humanity has paid too much attention to science and technology without limiting its discoveries to responsible uses and has left consciousness behind.

According to Hitler, if you repeat untrue information again and again without paying attention to the listeners, with the passage of time the listener will forget that what he is told is untrue, and it becomes truth. Thus untruth becomes accepted. There is an abuse of information in creating mass psychology in political, economical, scientific, social and religious fields.

In all political campaigns, policy and decision making processes, the repetition technique is used to convince the masses that their way is the right way. They use mass media, such as newspapers, fliers, magazines, radio talk shows, movies and television. The media has become very powerful in political policy and decision-making. This is true for the free world nations as well as socialist and communist countries.

Even corporations use this technique by having a well-known celebrity repeat advertisements again and again so they can sell their products, whether the celebrity uses them or not. All advertisements work on the principle of the influential nature of the subconscious mind. Millions of people lost their life's savings in the crash of the stock market. Their retirement funds became worthless. Stock analysts and investment firms hyped the stock market by providing the country with untrue information about the prospects, projected revenues and profits of corporations such as Enron, World Com and many others through various forms of media.

Whenever subjectivity is involved, informative knowledge is mostly untrue. The majority of humanity lives on informative knowledge as if it is the absolute truth and the food of life. At social events, gossip amongst guests center around information gathered from all kinds of media. Just as seen in the previous stock market example, anything based on something untrue will eventually fall apart.

Informative knowledge also plays a strong part in all organized religions where faith is deeply involved. Therefore there is a very high possibility of abuse. All preaching is based on the scriptures of the past. Neither the preachers nor their followers have personal, first hand experience. Since they are based on faith, they are told again and again with the same substance in various languages using different examples. After time, both the preachers and the listeners forget that what they have been told was not their personal experience, and they start believing as if it was.

The process of instilling faith starts at a very young age when the mind is a clean slate. A child is innocent and ignorant. During that time all informative knowledge about religion and living life is imparted again and again, and that becomes part of the life script deeply rooted in the subconscious mind. When a child turns into an adolescent, he is able to think and reason on his own. During this time, another set of information called doctrines and dogmas of hell and heaven are imposed and are used to build upon the life script. When an adolescent turns into a young adult, he has the ability to act upon his thoughts. He can make his own choices and decisions according to the life script written by others or can make new choices and decisions creating his own life script. The majority of humans live their lives according to a life script written by others. This creates conflicts between making new choices and decisions and the mindset of old beliefs and attitudes.

Most Islamic terrorists, for example, have been pounded with the idea of "Jihad" since childhood. They are willing to participate in any act of terrorism because they truly believe that if they die for their religion they are serving humanity and will go to heaven. They are willing to die for this belief.

Now is the time to explore a new kind of knowledge with innovative approaches to transmute, transform and transcend these mindsets from destructive to constructive.

Intellect and Intelligence
What is it in the human race that allows us to create the marvels of science and technology? Is it that human intellect and intelligence is in the pursuit of ideas, visions, and dreams of flying and reaching for the stars?

The Webster Dictionary definition of intellect is "perceiving and understanding; ability to reason; ability to perceive relations, differences and accept those differences; great mental ability".

How is intellect being developed? Your familiar senses receive information, which is processed through the brain and delivered to the mind (see figure "*The Process Flow Diagram of Intellect and Intelligence*").

The mind perceives this information, understands it and develops the perceptions. The mind is the flow of thoughts and feelings. Thoughts and feelings interact on those perceptions and questions: "What? How? And Why?" and thus creates the resonance of reasons. When these

Process Flow Diagram of Intellect and Intelligence

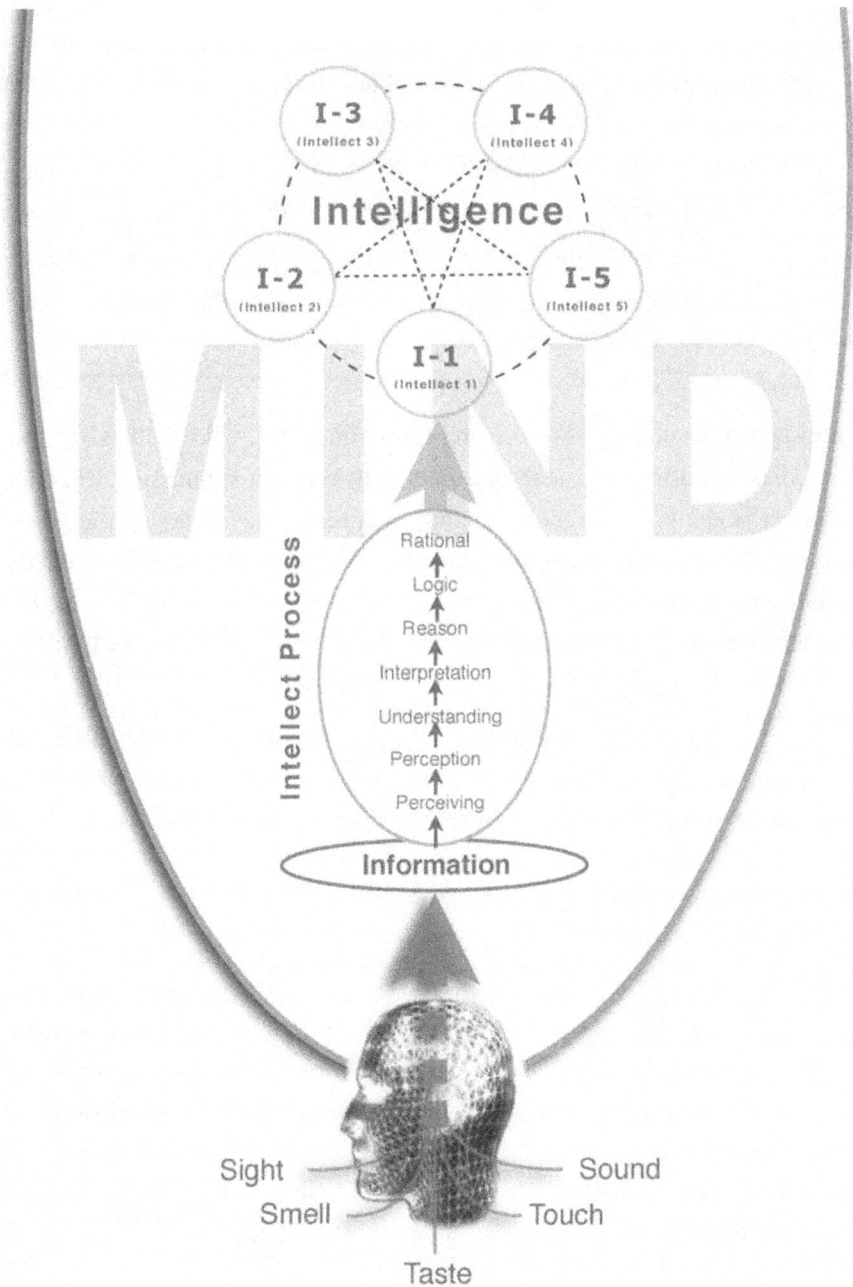

reasons are linked together, inductively or deductively, it is called logic. The mind conceives the logic and creates conception. The mind also develops fundamental reasoning on various issues or factual data, which is called rationality. This is the way intellect works.

The Webster Dictionary meaning of intelligence is: "a perception, discernment; the ability to learn or understand knowledge; mental ability; the ability to respond quickly and successfully to a new situation; use of faculty of reason in solving problems, directing conduct, etc. effectively."

Intelligence is analogous to the orchestra conductor, who synthesizes the melodies of various musical instruments to create a symphony, whereas intellect is analogous to the musician, each reading and playing the notes specific to his or her instrument. Intelligence is more focused on problem solving through connecting the dots, while intellect is more focused on knowing, finding, researching, discovering and understanding each of the data points or dots to be connected. Therefore, science is developed by intellectual pursuit while inventions and technology are developed by an intelligent pursuit of the application of science. Isaac Newton was more of a scientist whereas Thomas Edison was more of an inventor.

Let us journey through the history of humankind and explore the contribution of intellect and intelligence to humanity. What is their contribution to the magnificent discovery of the wonders of science and technology? To the change in the political systems from imperialism and kingdoms to modern democracy? To the union of humans by breaking the barriers of races, colors, caste, and classes? To the possibility of a higher standard of living? To the discovery of the sacredness of spirituality hidden in religious scriptures? Despite all these contributions, how did we still bring humanity closer to Global Suicide with weapons of mass destruction?

About four hundred years ago, the Orthodox Church believed that according to their scriptures, the earth was flat and that the sun revolved around it. The great Galileo, an astronomer and physicist, observed and measured the movements of the planets and realized that the earth was not flat and that it instead revolves around the sun. He developed the ability to understand the movements of the planets and perceive their relationships with each other, and through this he realized the differences between the Orthodox Church's beliefs and reality. His reasoning challenged the Catholic Church authorities in 1633 and he was arrested. He said, "putting me in jail and killing me won't make anything change. The facts remain the same. The facts are that the earth is round and the earth revolves around the sun". This started a major breakthrough within the general public and gave birth to a scientific revolution.

During the period of growth and evolution of intellect and intelligence, Francis Bacon, an English politician, philosopher and scientist said, "*If man will begin with certainties, he shall end in doubt; but if he will be content to begin with doubts, he will end in certainties.*" This still applies today, as we must doubt our current approaches and ask the hard questions to refine and evolve them.

Isaac Newton, physicist and mathematician, brought the power of observation and quantification to finding the laws of physics. In the 18th century, Benjamin Franklin used the power of "reason" and found electricity. In the 19th century, British physicist Michael Faraday combined logic and reason while applying the laws of nature to invent the electric motor. American physicist and inventor Thomas Edison electrified ideas using intellect and intelligence and invented more than 1,000 patents. In the 20th century, Albert Einstein, the physicist and astronomer, gave a new dimension and direction to intellect and intelligence with imagination and believed that "Imagination is more important than knowledge". He explored outer space and established the theory of relativity, which subsequently led to the development of nuclear energy. In the second half of the 20th century, the focus of intellect and intelligence shifted to the high tech revolution of computers, communication and the information age. This has created exponential progress in all dimensions and directions.

Since the beginning of recorded history there has been continuous growth of intellect and intelligence with the advancements of science and technology. There has been a shift in the power from organized religions and kingdoms to the people. People have become more intellectual and intelligent, better able to understand their rights and their powers. There have been constant revolts and revolutions all over the world, and as a result new political structures, such as democracy, socialism and communism, have evolved. These structures are based on intellectual idealism.

The industrialized nations (G8) created an abundance of wealth with the help of science and technology and the free enterprise system passing through the agricultural, industrial and high tech revolutions. They lifted the standard of living and quality of life to levels never seen before. This changed the entire fabric of society.

Intellect and intelligence are products of the human mind; the work of the human mind, the flow of thoughts and feelings, self or ego. The human mind can use intellect and intelligence for the betterment of humanity or can abuse it for greed, war or terrorism. Therefore, intellect and intelligence have many avenues of expression, from creativity to destruction, depending on the intent of the human mind.

The uses and abuses of intellect and intelligence depend upon how much objectivity and subjectivity is involved. When they are used objectively, they are a great benefit to humanity such as in the development of science. Generally science is a knowledge of finding, researching and discovering the laws of Mother Nature. Mother Nature includes the elements of earth, water, wind, fire and space as well as the mineral, plant, animal and human kingdoms. In observing and measuring Mother Nature, scientists are very objective. They observe without any pre-conditioned thoughts to derive the laws of Mother Nature. As a result, pure science and impure science have been developed. Pure sciences are those of physics, chemistry, and mathematics where maximum objectivity is involved. Impure sciences are about life and behavior where both objectivity and subjectivity are involved at various degrees. Impure sciences include medicine, psychology, sociology, politics, and economics.

Religious beliefs, on the other hand, are tremendously subjective. Therefore, there is a maximum abuse of intellect and intelligence in order to create fanatic mindsets. So, this second type of knowledge that we call intellect and intelligence is a double-edged sword. When used objectively, it can be a boon to society; however when used subjectively, it can be abused for selfish intentions and become a curse to humanity.

The current approaches of politics, diplomacy, military, economics and religion are based on the knowledge of intellect and intelligence. They are a mixed bag of objectivity and subjectivity. Objectively, we want to bring resolutions to the conflicts and eliminate terrorism so we can establish peace. Subjectively, we use politics and diplomacy as the means and methods in trying to defeat terrorism, which is based on ideological differences. Militarily, we use the power of Domination versus Dominion. Economically, we use the subjectivity of monetary power through benefits and losses. In addition, the insurmountable subjectivity of religious beliefs are deeply embedded in the subconscious mind.

The current use and knowledge derived from intellect and intelligence is not sufficient for finding resolutions to terrorism. We have to stretch further and reach for a knowledge that shows us how to work with the human mindset and belief systems in order to change the human intention that ultimately directs how intellect and intelligence is used.

Extra Sensory Perception (E.S.P.)
Extra sensory perception (E.S.P.) is the third type of knowledge. It has existed throughout the history of mankind but is not well recognized. Generally it is known as psychic knowledge. Every human being has the built-in abilities to perceive psychic phenomena, but few can recognize them and even fewer can develop those skills. Suppose you suddenly have a thought of a friend who you have long forgotten, and after a few minutes you receive a telephone call from that same friend. This psychic phenomenon is referred to as telepathy.

Senses are the doorways to life and knowledge. As discussed previously there are five familiar senses: sight, sound, smell, touch and taste. These familiar senses are called outer senses. The more sensitive these senses are, the more you experience life and expand your knowledge in all directions. The expansion of knowledge increases the information you receive, augments understanding and develops your intellect and intelligence, revealing the secrets of life.

The familiar outer senses are essentially antennas that receive different types of frequencies. We can also receive and perceive other types of frequencies directly through the brain and mind by increasing their sensitivity and receptivity. This is sometimes known as the 6th sense and is identified with special phenomena such as intuition, telepathy, clairvoyance, clairaudience, telekinesis and other psychic knowledge, which are all part of E.S.P. In the general public, there is a consensus that these abilities are available only to gifted or special people. In reality, these senses can be developed by anyone.

E.S.P. knowledge is based on trust, while science is developed by intellect and intelligence beginning with wonder and doubt and ending in certainty. Therefore, the people who are scientifically oriented find it difficult to understand E.S.P. despite the fact that the majority of inventions are created because of intuition. For example, Madame Curry solved an essential mathematical problem while sleeping. She physically solved the problem without remembering that she had done so the next day.

Interestingly, some people have been trained not to believe what they cannot see, touch or understand through reason. They cannot understand how the people living in primitive societies, such as the Amazon jungle, can develop the faculty of E.S.P. and apply it to survival, which we call basic instinct. Infact, there are many well-known people who were recognized for having E.S.P. Edgar Cayce was a psychic and clairvoyant during the 20th century. He gave more than 8,000 health readings while in trance. These readings consisted of diagnosis of disease or other health issues. He directed them to the doctor who would be able to help them and prescribe what was required to make them well. He also gave more than 4,000 life readings to people by uncovering their past lives – the lives that explained present dilemmas and conflicts. Even though he was a Christian and a Sunday school teacher, he accepted the existence of past lifetimes, reincarnation, and karmic laws.

We need someone like Edgar Cayce to locate the leaders of terrorist groups. The U.S. spends billions of dollars on the CIA, FBI, police departments, and defense for intelligence to find them. It seems that we are overly dependent on science and technology for finding both people and the solutions to our global illness. We need to think "outside the box" and go beyond the knowledge of intellect and intelligence and invest in the research of E.S.P. to develop the use of the psychic police, telepathic intelligence, clairvoyance and clairaudience in addition to satellite communications. Whatever science can do with equipment and technology, the human mind can add to with the help of these higher-tuned senses.

In summary, the first three types of knowledge are of the human mind. The first type of knowledge is the knowledge of information. The second type of knowledge is intellect and intelligence based on the information that has exponentially progressed. These two types of knowledge tremendously contribute to humanity where objectivity is involved. When subjectivity is involved, these two types of knowledge are double-edged swords. They are a boon to humanity when used to unite us, and a curse to humanity when used to divide us. The direction depends upon the intent of the human mind and human ego. Humanity can use this knowledge for betterment or abuse it for destruction. The third type of knowledge, E.S.P, is developed through the inner senses, and is still in its infancy, but will be further acknowledged in the 21st century.

Metaphysics
The Webster Dictionary meaning of Metaphysics is: "those things relating to external nature, after physics; the branch of philosophy that deals with the first principles and seeks to explain the nature of being or reality and the origin and structure of the world; is closely associated with a theory of knowledge; the theory or principles; subtle, perplexing or difficult reasoning".

The knowledge of Metaphysics is much more than the dictionary can convey. As described earlier, the brain exists within the space-time dimension and is therefore considered physical, however, the mind exists

46

beyond the space-time dimension because it cannot be touched or measured with a ruler or other physical measuring device and therefore is considered Metaphysical. The following are the dimensions and directions of Metaphysics for our path of Global Healing:

➢ Metaphysics is the knowledge of the human mind in its total complexity, which is generally known as "self" or "ego".

➢ Metaphysics is the knowledge of the body, mind, soul and spirit relationship.

➢ Metaphysics is understanding and knowing the dynamic process of the human mind.

➢ Metaphysics is the knowledge of transmuting, transforming and transcending negative emotions into positive emotions, negative ego into positive ego.

➢ Metaphysics is the pathway to spirituality.

➢ Metaphysics is the knowledge of how to consciously create reality.

In essence, Metaphysics is the knowledge that can teach us how to transform constrictive mindsets to constructive ones in an effort to overcome terrorism and create a better humanity.

Metaphysics is the knowledge of the human mind in its total complexity, which is generally known as the "self" or ego".
Just imagine the magnitude of this. Humanity consists of six billion people, each being a unique individual, unique in their physical form and individual in their personality or state of mind and ego. Each individual has their own beliefs, attitudes, thoughts, feelings, choices and decisions, which are always dynamically changing, fluctuating and shifting. Let us call these components raw materials on which each individual creates their reality using the crafting tools of desire, imagination and

expectation.

Each individual is in a different state of mind, at a different stage of needs and desires, and has a different level of knowledge. This creates the complexity of mind. In modern psychology, the mind is divided into three layers. The first layer is the conscious mind, which deals with the present and continuously makes choices and decisions while facing reality. The second layer is the subconscious mind, which is of the past where beliefs and attitudes are developed and the individual life script is written. The third layer is the unconscious mind and consists of all previous lifetimes. Whether you believe in previous lifetimes or not, there is still an unconscious mind.

<u>Metaphysics is the knowledge of the body, mind, soul and spirit relationship.</u>

The mind is located between the physical human body and Divine Energy which we shall refer to as "God/Goddess/All That Is". The physical body is connected to the mind through the brain. The brain receives information from the familiar senses and processes the information as programmed by the mindset and then passes it to the mind. The total (conscious, subconscious and unconscious) mind at the conscious level, responds to the information received through the brain during the awake state. The mind makes choices and decisions, and instructs the brain to act upon them through the hypothalamus gland. In turn, the brain instructs the body. Thus, there is an established body-mind relationship throughout life. In other words, the body is a gross mind and mind is a subtle body (see figure "*Metaphysics of Body-Mind-Soul-Spirit Relationship*").

The mind is continuously working through four states. The first state is "awake" when the conscious mind is working. The second state is

Metaphysics
of
The Body – Mind – Soul – Spirit Relationship

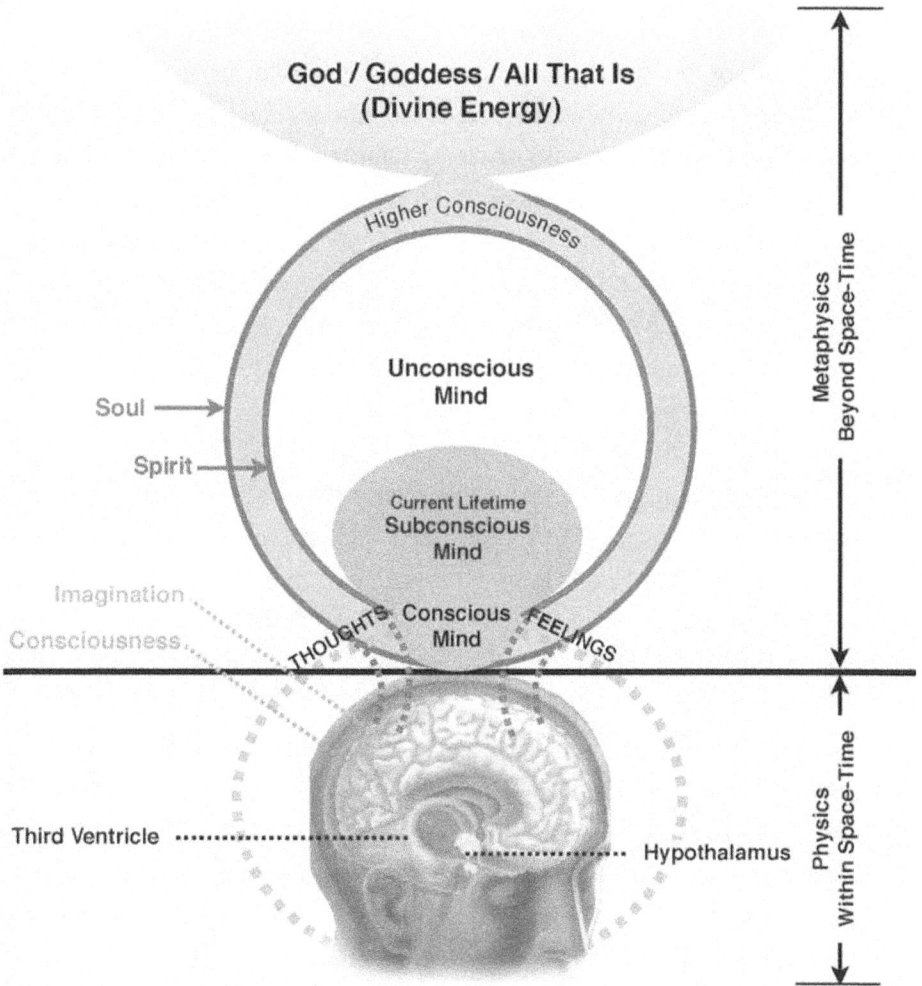

God / Goddess / All That Is
(Divine Energy)

Higher Consciousness

Unconscious
Mind

Soul →

Spirit →

Current Lifetime
Subconscious
Mind

Imagination

Consciousness

THOUGHTS Conscious FEELINGS
Mind

Metaphysics
Beyond Space-Time

Third Ventricle ··········

········· Hypothalamus

Physics
Within Space-Time

49

"asleep". In this state the subconscious and unconscious mind work through dreams and nightmares. The third state is a "deep sleep" when the mind almost enters a state of no-mind. The fourth state is where the mind is working but it is being observed objectively, the ego drops out and is totally witnessed by consciousness. As human senses are the doorway to life, the human mind with life, is the doorway to Divine Energy.

The mind, or the human ego, can work positively for personal growth to reach out and touch Divinity, or negatively for destruction of him or herself and others. Consciousness is required for the human mind to work positively. Consciousness has many levels such as attention, attentiveness, awareness, and on-going expansion. The expansion of consciousness comes from living in the present with the presence of the past and the future. According to modern Metaphysics, consciousness enters through the third ventricle of the human brain. Like a revolving door, it collects information throughout life.

The human mind deals with imagination, which is beyond space-time. Imagination is a very powerful tool used for consciously creating reality. All reality creation begins as an image in your imagination. Imagination is the doorway to the unfamiliar inner senses that link to the soul and spirit.

There are various mythological and religious concepts about the soul. In modern Metaphysics, the soul is eternal, it is never born and it never dies. The soul is a feminine energy where all conception of thoughts and ideas and all creativity happens. The Soul is always waiting to be found by the Spirit, which is masculine energy and has the ability to manifest the creativity of soul. The spirit is also in search of the Soul, like a man looking for a woman and a woman looking for a man. The spirit waxes and wanes, ebbs and flows. When a person is in a good mood and spirit, the person is a positive force, and during that time the spirit flows. When that force is depleted, the spirit wanes.

The soul and spirit together is your link to Divine Energy, which in organized religions, is called God. In modern Metaphysics, we refer to the Divine Energy as God/Goddess/All That Is, where God is masculine energy, Goddess is feminine energy, and combined together, they create All That Is. The human mind, self or ego, in this spiritual journey or pilgrimmage, uses the human body only as a vehicle.

<u>Metaphysics is the understanding and knowing the dynamic process of the human mind.</u>
Familiar senses deliver information to the brain, which in turn reports circumstances to the mind. The mind interacts with these circumstances and generates a new set of thoughts and feelings. Thoughts and feelings combine together creating emotions. The Metaphysical definition of emotion is "energy in motion". These emotions charged with energy are continuously changing, according to the state of mind, state of being and state of circumstances. Emotions can be generally classified in two groups: one is positive or expanding, and the other is negative or constricting as described on the next page.

Expanding and constricting emotions create the Metaphysical matrix of emotional energy (see figure *"Metaphysical Matrix of Emotional Energy"*). This makes a major contribution in the development of the human ego or self. Metaphysics is the knowledge of each emotion, how it is developed, what its causes and effects are, and what its implications are in the matrix of emotional energy.

Positive or Expanding Feelings/Emotions	Negative or Constricting Feelings/Emotions
I am good enough	I am not good enough
Trust	Fear
Love	Hate
Compassion	Indifference
Friendliness	Hostility
Friendship	Animosity
Gratitude	Ungrateful
Self-Love	Self pity
Inspirational/Appreciative	Comparison – Jealousy/Envy
Love	Martyr
Liveliness-Energy or Stimulation	Lifelessness-Depreciation
Challenge/Fun	Struggle/Stress
Fun & Joy	Duties & Obligations
Evaluating/Assessment	Judgemental/Conclusive
Freedom	Control
Dominion	Domination
With Grace	Under Force – Duress
Elegance	Hard Way
Concern	Anxiety
Caution	Worries
Non-Guilt	Guilt
Joy – Bliss	Dread
Caress – Tenderness	Rough – Rude
Merciful	Cruel
Being Limitless	Being Limiteed
Hopefulness – Enthusiasm	Depression
Wishfulness	Frustration
Pleasure	Pain
Playfulness	Suffering
Happiness	Unhappiness
Courage	Cowardice
Non-Conformity Adventure	Conformity

Metaphysical Matrix
of
Emotional Energy
(Thoughts & Feelings)

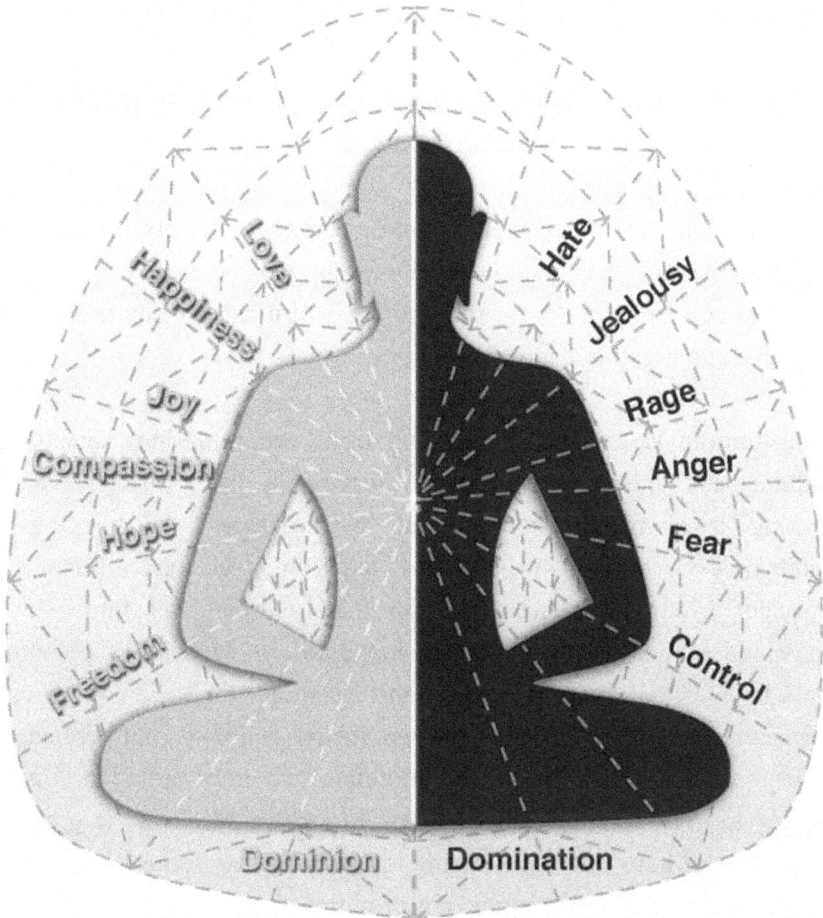

Metaphysics is the knowledge of transmuting, transforming and transcending negative emotions into positive emotions or the negative ego into the positive ego.

The positive ego, comprised of all positive emotions, is behind all growth and creativity and the negative ego, comprised of all negative emotions, is behind all struggle and destruction. Metaphysics is the knowledge of transmuting, transforming and transcending negative emotions into positive emotions.

Transmuting emotion is changing it from one emotion to another. The person who has a closed mind is stubborn and defensive. Once that person becomes open minded, the stubbornness is transmuted into determination and defensiveness into openness. Determination and openness are more useful and valuable for growth and creativity. Love is the most powerful energy for transmuting, and it can transmute any less effective emotion into a more useful one.

Transforming is changing something from one form into something different, an "unlike-form", where it intrinsically has a different value, making it more personally useful and valuable. For example, stubbornness and defensiveness combined with anger, hurt and fear are transmuted into determination and openness and then transformed into drive and action. Drive and action move something from its potential state to its actual state, which is transformation. Good intentions can transmute destructive emotions into productive emotions, but permanent change comes with dynamic manifestation and transformation. Being willing to give love and being willing to receive love are the greatest motivators of transformation. Being loved and letting someone love you is the most mystical and magical power of transformation.

Transcendence is changing something from one form to a higher octave form that is intrinsically and personally more valuable. It is the transformation of one state of mind into another. It allows you to be more of who you are. With transcendence, hate turns into love from the lower octave to the higher octave. It just happens without you always understanding how you get from the lower octave of hate to the higher octave of love.

Metaphysics is the pathway to spirituality.
The Webster Dictionary meaning of spirituality is, "spiritual nature, character, or quality, spiritual-mindedness". In Metaphysics, spirituality is the relationship with the Divine Energy, which many refer to as "God" however we have expanded that definition to "God/Goddess/All That Is". Every human being has a relationship with this Divine Energy. Even atheists have a relationship with God by not believing God exists. Theists have a relationship with God by believing in God either through blind faith, intellectual understanding, or through an on-going search because of some kind of personal experience.

Metaphysicians have a seeking relationship with God/Goddess/All That Is. They are not blind believers. They are open-minded to receiving information from the scriptures and other available sources. They are open to understanding spirituality using their intellect and intelligence and stretch beyond that to develop the courage to experiment, to personally experience their relationship. They are willing to risk themselves and enter into the unknown. At some point they are willing to gamble and become spiritual beings in their journey toward spirituality. In their journey, Metaphysics is a pathway of knowing their mind, self and ego, and understanding the body, mind, soul and spirit relationship.

The Metaphysical journey is transmuting, transforming and transcending negative emotions into positive emotions, changing the matrix of emotional energy to realign with Divine Energy. During this process, a person uses the power of the common senses of imagination and balance, and awakens the unfamiliar, inner senses of light, inner voice, movement, warmth and substance (see figure *"The Internet of Human Senses – Doorways to Life Part 2"*). These senses are the counterpart of the familiar/outer senses of sight, sound, smell, touch and taste.

Metaphysics is the knowledge of how to consciously create reality.

Metaphysics is the knowledge of the expansion of human consciousness. The first layer of consciousness is the conscious mind, which deals with the current situation in the awake state. The second layer is the subconscious mind where beliefs and attitudes are inscribed and all traits and habits are developed. The subconscious mind likes consistency, not changes. This is the main principle used to develop mass psychology. The father of modern psychology, Sigmund Freud, was right at that time when he said the seat of power is in the subconscious mind. However, as humanity has gained more self-awareness, the seat of power has now shifted from the subconscious mind to the conscious mind. The power of the conscious mind is in making choices and decisions continuously in the present to accomplish and achieve goals, visions and dreams of the future. Thus, there is a major shift in the paradigm of creating reality. The traditional paradigm is that the "past creates the present pushing us towards the future." The new paradigm is that the "future creates the present in the backdrop of the past."

Metaphysicians consciously create reality on the pathway to spirituality using the new paradigm in accordance with the Conscious Reality Creation Mantra:

> **I create my own reality, and**
> **I am responsible for what I am.**
> **I am the master of my destiny, and**
> **not a victim of fate.**

Internet of Human Senses
Doorways to Life – Part 2

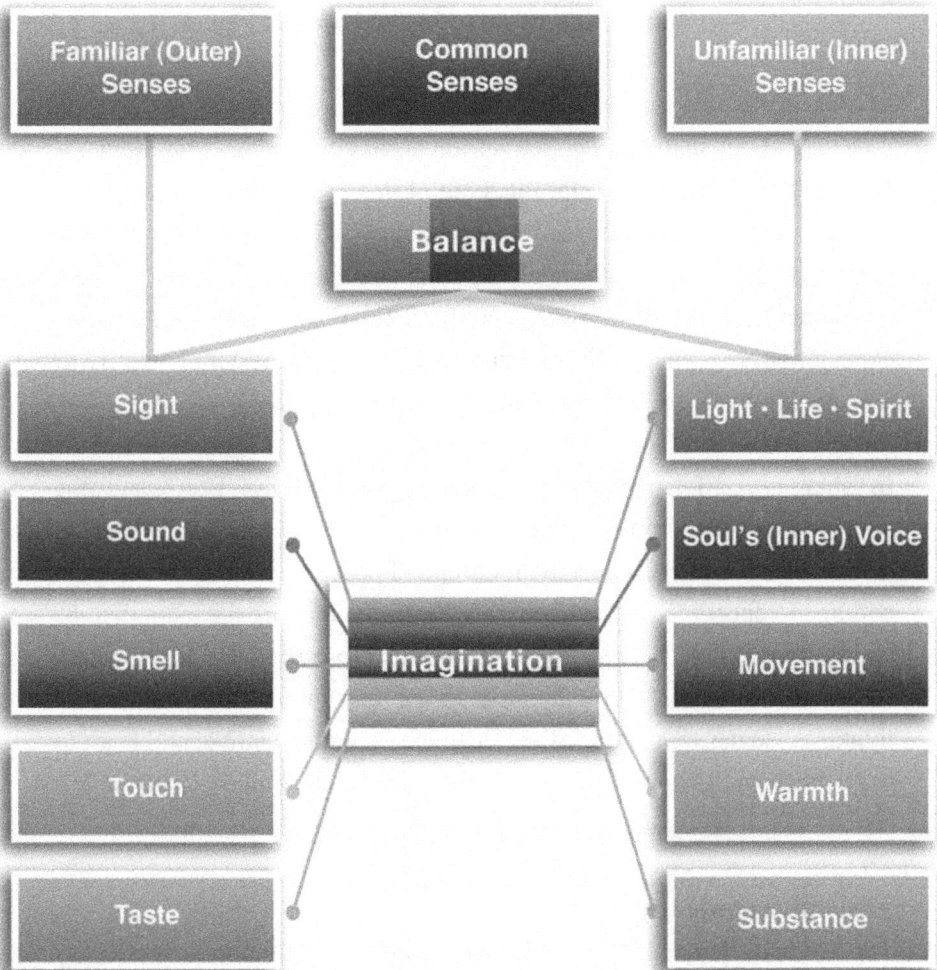

Familiar (Outer) Senses	Common Senses	Unfamiliar (Inner) Senses

Balance

Sight	Light · Life · Spirit
Sound	Soul's (Inner) Voice
Smell	Imagination	Movement
Touch	Warmth
Taste	Substance

The above mantra is out of responsibility. If we expand this mantra from the individual level to the community, national, and then global level, we say:

We (humanity at large) **create our own reality, and are responsible for what we are** (state of global illness). **We are the masters of our destiny** (creating Global Healing), **and not victims of fate** (Global Suicide).

Michelangelo saw the vision of Pieta in a large piece of marble. He dreamed about manifesting that vision into a sculpture. He used his hammers and chisels to sculpt Pieta out of this raw marble and his vision became real. Similarly, every human being is equally given the raw materials of beliefs and attitudes, thoughts and feelings, and choices and decisions. Each person is also given the tools of desire, imagination and expectation for consciously creating reality (see figure *"Raw Materials and Tools for Consciously Creating Reality"*).

In summary, Metaphysics is "Thinking Outside the Box" and the pathway to spirituality. The Metaphysician, on his pilgrimage to spirituality, has to create his own individual pathway. He has to have the courage to encounter the unknown. While encountering the unknown, he has to be creative in order to make further progress. He has to think differently and not allow himself to be conformed to conventional thinking. He has to be innovative, imaginative and inventive, and learn to draw from his dreams and visions in order to truly think "outside the box".

Absolute Knowledge
The Metaphysician (seeker) on his pilgrimage to spirituality, experiences glimpses of enlightenment and becomes a spiritual being (devotee). On his pilgrimage to enlightenment, the devotee keeps expanding his

Raw Materials & Tools
for
Consciously Creating Reality

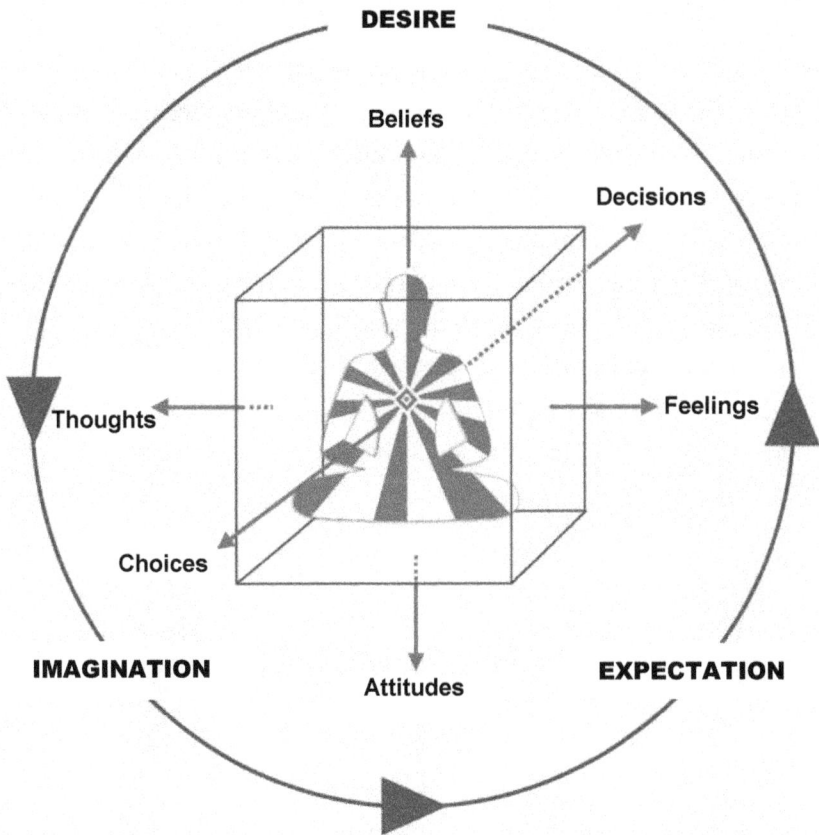

consciousness by observing his state of mind. At some point he breaks the identification with his state of mind and ego and turns into the total state of being. That state of being is enlightenment, a witness to his mind and body, where nothing remains to be learned and all that remains is knowledge, absolute knowledge. Absolute knowledge is the ultimate liberation; the total freedom of consciousness, which knows no limitations or impurity.

The current approaches to resolving terrorism and establishing world peace are derived from information, intellect and intelligence and based on "inside the box" thinking. These approaches are not working and humanity is heading towards Global Suicide. It is up to us to think "outside the box" by elevating our knowledge to the level of Metaphysics in order to learn how to change minds and mindsets so Global Healing can take place. We begin this task by diving deeper into the construct of the human mind in its total complexity.

Chapter 4

THINKING OUTSIDE THE BOX

Metaphysics is the knowledge of the human mind in its total complexity:

- ➤ What is the mind and its progression?
- ➤ What are the components of the mind?
- ➤ What are the layers of the mind and their functions?
- ➤ What is the development of the mind through the stages of life?
- ➤ What is the role of the mind in the body-mind-soul-spirit relationship?
- ➤ What is the relationship with the mind, self and ego?
- ➤ How is the mindset created and how can it be altered individually and collectively?

In order to understand the mind, we need to rely on something higher than the mind, and that is consciousness - the state of awareness that you are being aware. The Metaphysician's approach to understanding the mind is through the process of meditation. A Metaphysician is a spiritual scientist who focuses on exploring and observing the mind using meditation to seek answers from within rather than outside as a traditional scientist does with physical instruments and devices.

Generally, a Metaphysician begins this journey by entering into a relaxed state of mind and eventually progresses into a meditative state by passing through various states of mind. When someone first begins the practice of meditation, they pass through a confused state of mind. In this state, thousands of thoughts and images are running in all directions and dimensions creating a wide variety of feelings from sadness to joy and from pain to love. The meditator remains unfocused and resists confronting their own thoughts and feelings. These thoughts could be feelings of the past or desires of the future. They could be dreams, nightmares, visions or unknown images that can be either pleasant or troubling, beautiful or ugly.

With practice, meditation progresses to a contemplative state of mind. The Webster Dictionary definition of contemplation is, "the act of looking at or thinking about something intently; the act of mind in considering with attention; study; consideration." The Metaphysical definition of contemplation is "funneling attention to channel thoughts on a certain subject matter from various perspectives." For example, when a college student prepares for a test in physics, he channels all thoughts related to physics, and he avoids entertaining other thoughts. As his contemplation progresses, he logically sequences his thoughts and puts all the pieces together to gain a greater understanding. Then he develops intellect and intelligence.

With further practice the meditator enters a state of complete concentration. The Webster Dictionary definition of concentration is: "fixed or close attention". The Metaphysical definition of concentration is "the condensing of focus onto a certain subject matter". For example, when a driver is driving a car in extremely bad weather conditions, he remains totally focused on the road, the steering wheel and the brake pedal. He does not listen to the radio, talk with passengers or entertain any other thoughts in his mind.

The seeker in his continuous pursuit of spirituality then enters into the meditative state of mind. The Webster Dictionary definition of meditation is, "a thinking over, serious contemplation; the act of meditating; close or continued thought; the turning or revolving of a subject in the mind; mental reflection." The Metaphysical meaning of meditation is much more than that. Meditation is the process of expanding one's consciousness through continual condensing of their focus until one becomes detached or unidentified with their own thoughts, feelings or images and in turn becomes an observer of them. Through continuous progress, "observing" turns into "witnessing" and the Metaphysician turns into a spiritual being and becomes enlightened when he becomes a total witness. This occurs when the ego has dropped out allowing the mind to enter into a state of no-mind.

In essence, this is a Metaphysician's journey from confused-mind to no-mind. In the beginning, the meditator remains identified with his thoughts and feelings, however, with practice he gradually develops his consciousness, observing thoughts, feelings and images coming from all directions and from time dimensions of past, present, future or the unknown. With continuous practice, he starts detaching himself from his thoughts and feelings and becomes an observer of them along with other images through the expansion of consciousness. He now becomes a Metaphysician, or in other words, a spiritual scientist.

Components of Mind

The Metaphysician uses the knowledge of information, intellect, intelligence and E.S.P. and stretches past them to know the mind by using the mind itself. So, the Metaphysician looks beyond the mind by involving consciousness – the state of awareness that he is being aware - to know the mind better. In other words, the Metaphysician plays with consciousness. He expands his consciousness by having it increase, spread, augment and reveal itself. The expanding consciousness helps the Metaphysician to understand the complexity of how the mind works and functions. This is done by exploring each emotion in connection with the matrix of emotional energy. For instance, jealousy is developed through comparison, unhealthy competition and forming feelings of deprivation. Then jealousy is expressed in daily activities through feelings of anger, control, sabotage, and in some cases, through violence.

Human beings receive information from the outer world by the five familiar senses of sight, sound, smell, touch and taste. This information is processed through the brain and passed to the human mind. The brain and mind work together intricately. The brain is part of physics, within the space-time dimension and the mind is part of Metaphysics, beyond the space-time dimension. Suppose you are driving a car on the highway, receiving information from billboards, highway signs, radios, CD players, conversations with passengers, drinking coffee or eating food, talking on a cell phone, watching the scenery, the weather and smelling fragrances. All this information is delivered to the brain. The brain processes all information according to the individual's mindset. Only information that is given meaning, significance and value by the mindset is processed. This in turn generates thoughts and feelings.

The major components of the human mind are thoughts, feelings and images. Thoughts recognize, acknowledge and identify feelings. Suppose you are hungry. There is a feeling of hunger but that feeling only exists if it is recognized by a thought. Therefore, thoughts and feelings are generated simultaneously. When thoughts and feelings are coupled together, we call them emotions, or energy-in-motion as previously described. These emotions are part of the human mind, which is essentially a flow of thoughts and feelings, and the emotional intensity can range from very low to very high.

The space dimension consists of length, width and depth and the time dimension consists of past, present and future. For linear understanding, the time dimension can be grouped into three categories. First is chronological time, which includes the past, present and future such as the years 2005, 2006, 2007, etc. and is perceived to be the same by all people. The second is called psychological time. Psychological time is personalized to the individual and shrinks or expands depending on an individual's state of mind. If an individual is engrossed in an activity, then time shrinks. If an individual is bored and not stimulated, then time expands. The third is metaphysical or spiritual time, which is timeless time, where time is revealed as an illusion.

When an individual goes into an altered state of mind, or out of body, time becomes an illusion where past, present and future merge and become one - timeless time. Ego disappears and the mind enters a state of no-mind. The individual is in the state of timelessness, limitlessness and egolessness. Individuals experience this state of mind when they are in a deep sleep and seekers experience this by consciously going into deep meditation.

When emotions are given greater meaning, significance and value, they are contained in receptacles, which we call memories. Memories consist of past events and incidents; therefore they are part of the subconscious and unconscious mind.

Imagination does not occupy space-time, it is beyond space-time and therefore Metaphysical. Imagination is also a common sense, commonly given to everybody. If you close your eyes, you can imagine a six-foot tall human being and you can expand that image to a sixty-foot tall giant, or contract the image to a six-inch dwarf. Usually, images of the physical universe are received through the eyes using the sense of sight. The eyes in turn transmit images to the occipital lobe of the brain. The brain and mind work together and store images in the mind. Thus, there is a body-mind relationship in receiving and storing the images from the physical universe. Although millions of images are received through the eyes, or the sense of sight, few are given meaning and significance by human emotions, thoughts and feelings. Those images that are given meaning and significance become part of the subconscious mind, which is part of the current lifetime.

The human mind also has the ability to conjure up new images through the power of visualization, which we call dreaming. Dreaming can be day-dreaming, lucid dreaming and/or night dreaming. During the sleep state, the subconscious mind, unconscious mind and the future self - that which you expect or want to become - display images. These images may be in a logical sequence of events, projected futures, or random where they don't make any sense. Images have their own language. They can be pleasant dreams or scary nightmares.

Moreover, the soul communicates through images, since images are the language of the soul. All creativity comes out of the power of imagination, which lies in what a Metaphysician refers to as the Imaginal Realm or the Realm of Images accessed through one's imagination. Before anything comes into reality, it must first exist as an image, and only then can it be manifested into reality. Even Albert Einstein recognized this when he said, "Imagination is more important than knowledge."

Layers of the Mind and Their Functions
The human mind has four layers. The first is the conscious mind, which deals with the current activities, events and incidents. The conscious mind has three main functions. The first function is the compelling force to confront and deal with the reality of current activities, events and incidents to satisfy needs. The second function is the propelling force to make choices and decisions to accomplish desires, goals, dreams and

visions. The third function is the driving force of knowing the mysteries of life and the mysteries of the universe.

The second layer of the human mind is the subconscious mind of the current lifetime. In the journey of human life from birth to death, the mind constantly develops through the experiences and incidents of life creating beliefs, attitudes and memories. These are stored in the subconscious mind.

The third layer is the unconscious mind of previous lifetimes or the unknown realm. When an infant is born, he brings beliefs, attitudes and some memories from either a past lifetime, if you believe in past lifetimes, or from an unknown realm. Therefore, each individual is unique. Each individual has a unique personality, unique personal traits, personal vocations, personal likings and dislikings, personal pursuits, desires and dreams and way of living. All of these characteristics are part of the unconscious mind. Metaphysically, the unconscious mind is vaster than the physical universe. Exploration of the unconscious mind will become a significant focus in the 21st century just as the exploration of space and the physical universe was in the 20th century.

The fourth layer of the human mind is the higher consciousness or higher-self who knows the journey of your soul from the beginning and is ready to guide you in your pilgrimage back toward the sweet home of Divinity.

In summary, the conscious mind, in combination with the subconscious and unconscious mind, is always dynamic and constantly generating thoughts and feelings by interacting with current events, incidents and relationships in life. Through this process, the mind creates a matrix of emotional energy of thoughts and feelings. This matrix is the emotional or psychic body consisting of the conscious mind, subconscious mind and unconscious mind. This emotional body is always in flux as a dynamic process and the matrix has a wide range of complex emotions interacting with each other constantly and can be classified into positive or expanding emotions and negative or constricting emotions.

Metaphysically all emotions in the emotional body are functions that are expressed and reflected in day-to-day life during a myriad of activities. For example, if a person is angry, he can express his anger through shouting, screaming, throwing objects, or physically or emotionally hurting people in any number of other ways. However, when the anger is not physically expressed, then it is reflected through facial expressions, sound of his voice and/or psychosomatic diseases. According to Metaphysics, the root cause of cancer is putrefied anger. Physicians may be able to remove the symptoms by chemotherapy, but cannot heal the patient because the cause lies in the mind, not in the body. The body reflects the effects of the cause. The emotional body constantly expresses or reflects itself in both the awake state of mind through daily activities and sleep state of mind through dreams and nightmares.

Development of the Mind Through the Stages of Life
The matrix of emotional energy creates the mindset of a human being. According to the mindset, a human being perceives and develops perception and conceives and creates conception. A mindset is like a filter on a camera. The poet Emerson said, "If you look through dark glasses, everything is gloomy. If you look through rosy glasses, everything is rosy."

To truly defeat terrorism and achieve Global Healing, we need to understand the development of the human mindset, which in turn helps us understand the terrorist mindset (see figure "*Development of Mindset*").

Development of Mindset

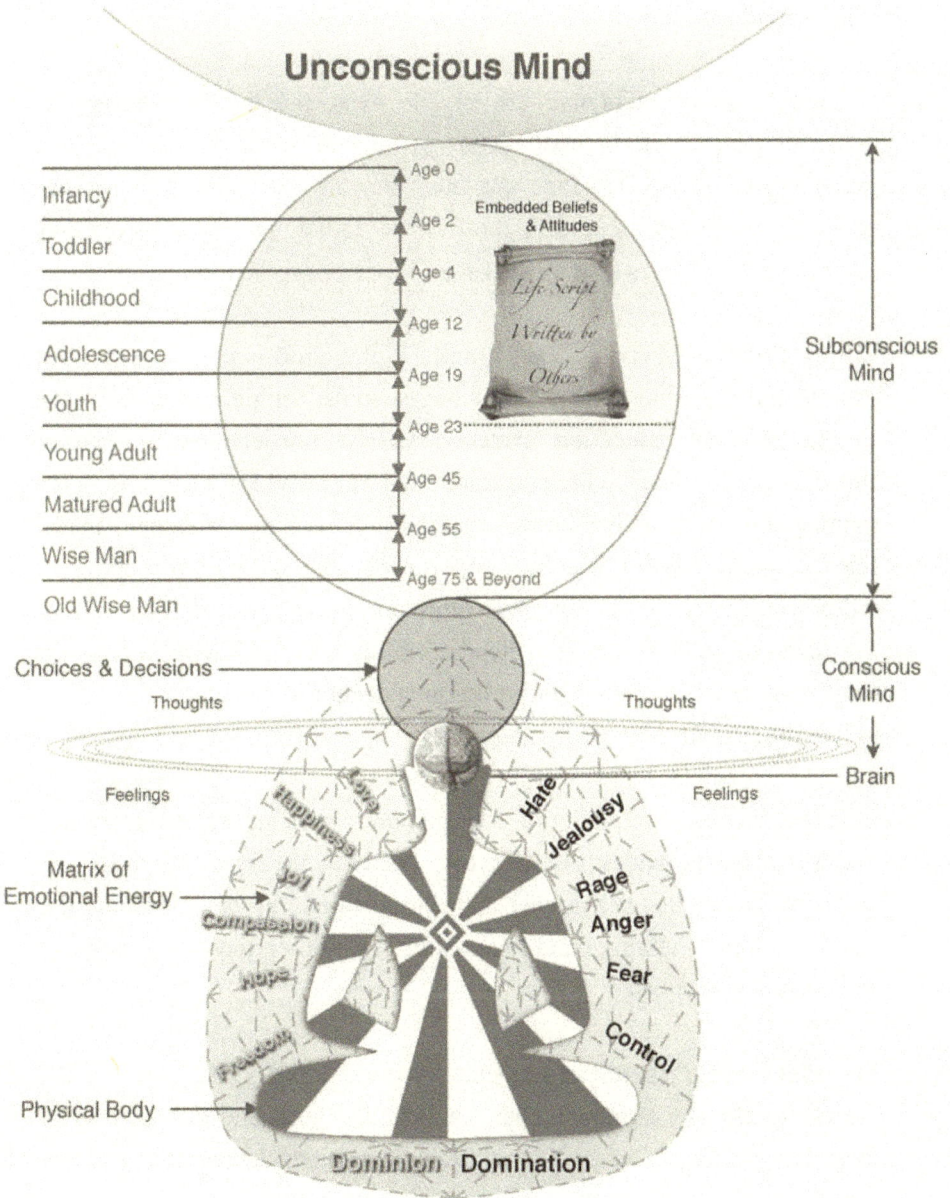

Unconscious Mind

Age 0
Infancy
Age 2
Toddler
Embedded Beliefs
& Attitudes
Age 4
Childhood
Age 12
Life Script
Adolescence
Written by
Age 19
Others
Youth
Age 23
Young Adult
Age 45
Matured Adult
Age 55
Wise Man
Age 75 & Beyond
Old Wise Man

Subconscious
Mind

Choices & Decisions

Conscious
Mind

Thoughts   Thoughts

Brain

Feelings   Feelings

Love
Happiness   Hate
Jealousy
Joy
Matrix of
Emotional Energy   Rage
Compassion   Anger
Hope   Fear
Freedom   Control

Physical Body

Dominion Domination

When an infant is born he or she is totally innocent and works through unfamiliar senses trusting the existence for survival. After a few weeks, the infant becomes aware of him or herself and the familiar senses of sight, sound, smell, touch, and taste start developing.

When the infant enters into the terrible twos, the familiar senses are totally developed. He is totally aware of himself, separates from mother psychologically and develops the "me, me, me" attitude. During this period between ages 2 and 4, the mother, father, brothers, sisters and other family members start writing the life script for the toddler.

During childhood between ages 4 and 12, the child is taught by his/her parents and siblings, family, neighbors, schools, religions, societies and nations through education systems, sports, music, arts and other curricular activities. The education system provides the child with training and informative knowledge through reading, language, math, science, social studies, practical experiments and vocational training in order to deal with the tangible physical world. At the same time, organized religion and family members teach the child about intangible subjective beliefs such as God, religion and faith, dos and don'ts of how to live life, morals and values and more.

During childhood "me, me, me" expands into "mine, mine, this is mine", like a warrior expanding his territory. Between the ages 9 and 12, the child recognizes that the mother is trying to satisfy all his needs and the child develops a helping hand in assisting his mother and father, siblings and friends in that task.

The child becomes an adolescent at approximately the age of 12. Hormones change, attraction changes, boys like girls and girls like boys, there is a surge of energy. The adolescent starts developing his own thinking and begins making his own choices and decisions. However, adolescent thinking is influenced by schools, peer groups, religions, parents, society, country, other associations and environments. The education system provides objective lessons to develop the second kind of knowledge, intellect and intelligence, and teaches how to apply them in the physical world and in real life. The education system also provides subjective teachings, psychology, sociology, discipline, and ethics.

At the age of 20, the adolescent enters into youth. During this period, the youth has tremendous energy to do many things. He has dreams of becoming a doctor, lawyer, engineer, policeman or fireman, but he does not have the ability to manifest those dreams. At this age he starts preparing for the real world in which he will create his own destiny, where he can manifest his dreams and visions.

Before the youth becomes a young adult at the age of 23, his life script is written by others. Their beliefs and attitudes have already been established in the young adult's life script and become a part of his subconscious mind. These beliefs and attitudes are:

- ➢ I am a Christian. I am Jewish. I am Islamic. I am Hindu. I am Buddhist.
- ➢ I am American. I am Canadian. I am European. I am Asian. I am Palestinian. I am Israeli.
- ➢ I am a Democrat. I am a Republican.
- ➢ I am a communist. I am a Socialist. I am a Capitalist.
- ➢ I am white. I am brown. I am black.
- ➢ I am handsome. I am average. I am beautiful. I am ugly.
- ➢ I am rich. I am poor.

The young adult continues the journey of life. Practice is over, he is now a player and actor on the world stage. He comes across two extreme options. The first option is to become a player of a life script written by others or dictated by beliefs and attitudes of the past embedded within the subconscious mind. The second option is to rewrite a life script according to his own dreams and visions, choices and decisions and become the author and player on the world stage. He has to make his own choices and decisions to create his own destiny. Between these two major options there are thousands of possibilities. Each human being develops his own choices and decisions. The mindset remains continuously in flux and dynamism with the passage of life from young adulthood until death.

The beliefs and attitudes of life are deeply embedded in the subconscious mind where all habits, good or bad, virtues and vices are developed. The subconscious mind likes consistency and resists changes, no adventures. It is generally said that the subconscious mind is eight times more powerful than the conscious mind, however the conscious mind can use the power of choice as leverage against the subconscious mind.

Choices and decisions are made in the conscious mind and are continual. The conscious mind has a special ability to make new choices and decisions while the subconscious mind does not have that ability. There is a balance of power between the subconscious mind and the conscious mind. The conscious mind has the ability to rewrite the life scripts written in the subconscious mind and change embedded beliefs and attitudes.

The continuous interaction between the choices and decisions of the conscious mind and the beliefs and attitudes of the subconscious and unconscious mind generate thoughts and feelings. These thoughts and feelings activate the brain and are expressed through activities in day-to-day life in creating reality. In reality creation, individually and collectively, there are three sets of raw materials available to everybody. The first set is the beliefs and attitudes of the subconscious and unconscious mind. The second set is the thoughts and feelings, which are being constantly generated. The third set is the choices and decisions of the conscious mind.

In crafting reality from raw materials, tools are required. The basic tools available to everybody are desire, imagination and expectation. Michelangelo saw the vision of Pieta in a big marble stone and sculpted it by using the tools of hammers and chisels. Similarly, each human being sculpts his own reality physically, mentally, emotionally and spiritually, by using the tools of desire, imagination and expectation on the raw materials given to them as shown in the *"Raw Materials & Tools for Consciously Creating Reality"* diagram in the previous chapter.

The majority of human beings live their lives according to the life script written by others. However, a small percentage of humanity rewrites their life script by creating new choices and decisions based on what they want to become. By rewriting their life script, they change their beliefs and attitudes of the subconscious mind. This small percentage of people are successful in accomplishing their desires, and they become leaders for the rest of humanity. The majority of humanity is busy satisfying their basic needs of survival, security, and belonging, and they don't have much time to see the larger picture of the Global Family as a whole and which direction it is heading. They are being influenced by repetitive messages from television, radio, newspaper, books and their leaders, which in turn creates mass psychology. They give their power to leaders who make choices and decisions on their behalf. This mass psychology is deeply rooted in the collective unconscious. Their mindsets resist new choices and decisions and make it difficult for them to think "outside the box".

Beliefs and attitudes of the subconscious mind play a vital role in life. Beliefs do not like change, they like consistency. Beliefs engrained in childhood are deeply embedded in the subconscious mind. For understanding, beliefs can be divided into two types: objective belief and subjective belief. Objective belief deals with the tangible world, which you can see, hear, smell, touch and taste through the five familiar senses. Subjective belief deals with the intangible world such as believing or disbelieving in God, believing in heaven and hell, likes and dislikes, relationships and personal prejudices.

As far as objective beliefs are concerned, the first two types of knowledge – namely, information, intellect and intelligence - have done a wonderful job in the 20th century by contributing to the development of science and technology. Objective beliefs can be altered, changed or modified by practical experiments of science and technology.

As far as subjective beliefs are concerned, the knowledge of information, intellect and intelligence has developed psychology, behavior science, political science, social science, sociology, socio-psychology, psychotherapy and psychiatry. However, all these subjects have been developed by using information, empirical data, reason, logic, logical sequence, and rationality. These subjects are not sufficient to bring a resolution of conflicts created by subjective beliefs, especially with regard to the war on terrorism.

If we journey through the 20th century, the major conflicts, revolutions and wars have happened because of the conflicts over subjective beliefs.

The philosopher Karl Marx came up with the political theory called communism. Although not originally intended by Marx, the communist theory has since evolved to state that matter is, there is no God and everyone is equal, therefore, wealth should be reallocated by equal distribution. Lenin applied this version of the theory and brought communism to Russia through the Russian Revolution. Stalin further

76

abused the theory and created massacres of intellectuals. After the Second World War, humanity passed through the cold war period accelerating and piling up military arsenals with nuclear weapons of mass destruction. Humanity realized that it was heading towards Global Suicide unless this behavior stopped. There was the fall of the Berlin Wall between the east and west and the breakdown of the USSR. Talks and treaties of disarmament between Russia and the USA continued, and the cold war period ended. However, the hidden residual currents of communism still prevail today through China, North Korea, and Cuba.

Hitler imposed the belief in Germany that the Aryan race is the supreme race and should rule the world. With this belief, he started the Second World War in Europe, and millions of people were killed. Japan followed the same principles of supremacy and attacked Pearl Harbor. The USA responded declaring war on Japan and eventually dropping atomic bombs on Hiroshima and Nagasaki forcing Japan to surrender. Humanity learned a big lesson. If we continue with nuclear weapons we are heading toward Global Suicide.

The above conflicts and wars were resolved by Domination, using power of military strength, however today we have different levels of conflicts and wars. This war involves terrorism created by the religious belief system of "Jihad". Terrorism has become a cancer spreading throughout humanity, but cannot be healed by the chemotherapy and radiation treatment methods of Domination. The leaders, who are trying to win the war on terrorism, are using political, diplomatic, military, economic and religious approaches through their own subjectivity. This creates perpetual subjective conflict without bringing any resolutions, keeping us on the path toward Global Suicide.

Understanding the Mindsets of Terrorists
Terrorism is based on conflicts of subjective beliefs. These subjective

beliefs are religious beliefs of "Jihad", dying for the Islamic religion, and are deeply embedded in the subconscious mind. These beliefs are fanatic beliefs and those that practice them are fanatics. According to the Webster Dictionary, a fanatic is defined as "a person who has excessive and unreasonable enthusiasm or zeal".

> *The Islamic military conquered the city of Alexandria in 640AD. It had the biggest library of that time, storing all the books and knowledge of various civilizations written by Aristotle, Plato and others. Caliph Omar, an army leader approached the librarian with his right hand holding a sword and his left hand holding the Quran. He asked the librarian to accept the Quran and become Islamic, otherwise he would kill her and burn down the library. He said the Quran is right and these books in the library were wrong. The librarian said 'I don't know the Quran, how can I say anything about it? The Quran may be right or may not be, but I know about these books. I can discuss them with you.' Caliph said 'No discussion. I say the Quran is right. Either you accept it or not.' He killed the librarian and burned the library. The fire lasted for several months and mankind lost the knowledge of Atlantis and many other civilizations. Caliph was a fanatic. He knew in his heart that he didn't know what was right or what was wrong. So to cover up his ignorance, he enforced his belief with excessive and unreasonable enthusiasm.*

Among all subjective beliefs, religious subjective beliefs are the most deeply rooted in the collective unconscious. Religious beliefs are about the relationship with God or Divine Energy. In these kinds of beliefs, both the relationship with God, and God are intangible. In other subjective beliefs, such as political idealism, the relationship with ideals of communism, socialism and democracy are intangible, but the people who believe in them are tangible. The idea of supremacy of race is intangible but people who believe in that are tangible. Therefore, political idealism and supremacy of race are changed through the tangible processes of war, negotiations, treaties, progress and prosperity.

The majority of humanity believes in God. Theists have been influenced by organized religions in establishing their relationship with God. These organized religions include Christianity, Islam, Judaism, Hinduism, Buddhism, Jainism, Taoism, Shintuism and others. Each religion has many denominations. Children are born into families that can be liberal, conservative, orthodox/ultra-conservative or fanatic in their religious beliefs. Children who are born into ultra-conservative and fanatic families are rigorously taught religion throughout childhood. These teachings come from the religious scriptures interpreted by religious teachers called priests, mullahs, rabbis, gurus or monks.

> *A child's mind begins as a "clean slate". Teachers write their religious scripts on this "clean slate" repeatedly, for years. During adolescence, children are indoctrinated with religious interpretations of scriptures instilling the fear of hell and greed of heaven. Both hell and heaven are imaginative and are intangible.*

When adolescents become adults, they carry their subjective religious belief script written by others. Many of them receive an education through schools, colleges and universities. They receive degrees in science, math, and art and continuously change their objective beliefs, but the subjective religious belief system usually remains the same because it is so deeply ingrained in their subconscious mind. They carry the fanatic psychology of religious beliefs irrespective of their education.

These religious fanatics believe that dying for their religion is the purpose of their lives. When they die, they expect to go to heaven, and believe heaven is very beautiful. These fanatics are indoctrinated with hate, hating all who do not believe in their religion. They turn into terrorists, willing to perform and die according to their religious script interpreted by others. They are aware that the terrifying acts of violence can create a field of fear upon which they can force their beliefs and will upon others to accept their way of thinking with their terms. Again, the mindset is either my way or the highway. There is no discussion, dialogue or negotiation. How to undo or change their mindset is the Metaphysical challenge for humanity.

Formation of Terrorists' Organizations

Terrorist organizations have fanatic mission statements. Their objectives are accomplished by performing and spreading terrorist acts. Like regular organizations there are three major departments. The first is the marketing department, which markets their religious beliefs, interpreted by vested interest groups such as Ayatollahs and Mullahs. These Ayatollahs and Mullahs indoctrinate children and adolescents through their own interpretation of the scriptures in religious schools called Madrasas. They also recruit youngsters who are helpless, hopeless and have nothing to lose and give them value through the religious beliefs (see photographs of Al Queda in *Madrasa and Campus Area*).

The second is the production department. In this case, the production department trains the indoctrinated children, adolescents, and recruited youngsters to perform terrifying acts of violence.

The third is the finance department, which supports the whole operation of recruiting youngsters, running Madrasas and the training classes to perform terrorist acts. This financing is done through charities under the name of religion.

The leaders of these organizations, recruiters, trainers and financiers

Madrasa and Campus Area
Development of Mindset

"I had a question for the students: Who wants to see Osama bin Laden armed with nuclear weapons? Every hand in the room shot up. The students laughed and some applauded."

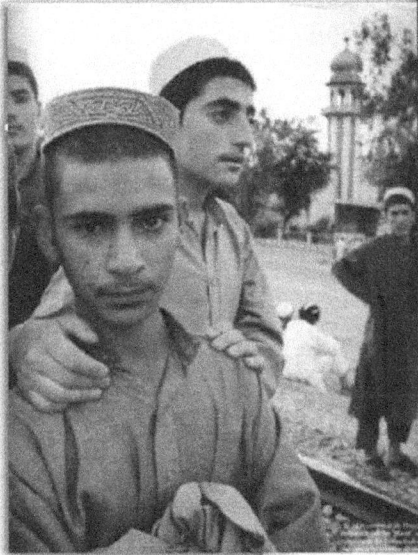

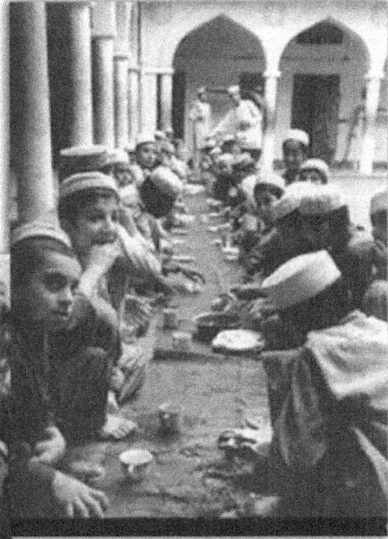

"On Campus at the Haqqania madrasa, which has 'placed' more students in the Taliban leadership than any other school in the world"

Photographs and quotations are from the New York Times Magazine, June 25, 2000 / Section 6.

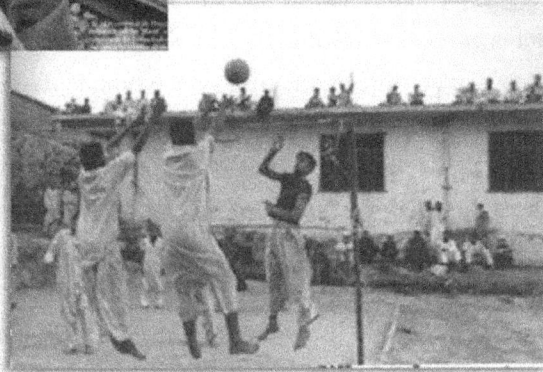

81

have a common goal and vested interests. They want to remain in control and have the power to rule in order to fulfill their subjective, religious and fanatic beliefs without any discussion, dialogue or negotiation. These terrorist organizations spread terrorists throughout populations of humanity and create violent acts to create a field of fear. Daily life becomes paralyzed. There is no economical, political, cultural, or creative growth. All military, political, economic and diplomatic moves become less and less effective. We, humanity at large, have created this, and we are responsible for it. So, we have to be imaginative, innovative and inventive in our attempt to find new ways to resolve these conflicts by changing the mindset of terrorists.

Mythology, along with the history of mankind, reveals that great people always thought "outside the box" to change the course of human consciousness, civilizations, literature, arts, music, philosophy, science and technology, and entrepreneurship. Both eastern and western mythology teach us lessons relating to the journey of the human soul in pursuit of spirituality while on the path of Metaphysics. The history of mankind teaches us the lessons about the rise and fall of human ego on the path of Domination.

Many spiritual leaders and mystics, western or eastern, northern or southern, such as King David, King Solomon and Moses of Judaism; Jesus Christ of Christianity; Mohammed of Islam; Ram, Krishna, and several others of Hinduism; Buddha of Buddhism; Mahaveer of Jainism; Lao-T-Se of Taoism; Rumi of Sufism; Zen masters of Japan and many others listened to their soul's call to adventure. They developed the courage to break the bonds of traditional thinking and pursued spirituality. They came across mystical experiences, liberated their people, found their spiritual path, and created a map used for the evolution of consciousness.

THINKING OUTSIDE THE BOX

Great Political leaders, such as Abraham Lincoln, Mahatma Gandhi, Martin Luther King, and Nelson Mandela listened to their soul's call to adventure and developed the courage of thinking "outside the box" while they pursued their dreams and visions. They became the mapmakers for humanity at large to listen to the soul's calls for adventure and free people from discrimination, injustice, misery and Domination.

All the great scientists, astronomers, mathematicians, inventors and technologists such as Galileo; Isaac Newton, Benjamin Franklin, Michael Faraday, Thomas Edison, Charles Darwin, Madame Currie, Albert Einstein and several others of the 20th century, listened to their soul's call to adventure and developed the courage of thinking "outside the box". They pursued their dreams and visions and discovered the laws of nature. They developed science and technology that have been a boon to humanity. They took humanity from the agricultural revolution to the industrial revolution, then to the high-tech revolution of computers and the information age.

In the 20th century, humanity paid too much attention to developing science and technology and not enough attention to human relations and the sustainability of the planet. Humanity looked to science and technology for the cure of all ills including the defeat of terrorism. Yet, "science and technology" is a double-edged sword, it cuts both ways. It is a boon and a curse depending upon how we use it or abuse it. If we use it with an evolved consciousness then it is a boon. Otherwise it is a curse.

Thinking "inside the box" is the expansion of the current knowledge of information, intellect and intelligence and then the modification of conventional politics, diplomacy, military, United Nations' resolutions, negotiations, treaties, and cease-fires.

To think "outside the box" is to stretch beyond the knowledge of information, intellect and intelligence and explore new, imaginative, innovative and inventive approaches such as enchanted wisdom.

> *Now is the time*
> *to cut the edge of thinking inside the box.*
> *TO RISK*
> *the known, the familiar and comfortable ideas,*
> *the mass psychology of the collective mind,*
> *that believes the approaches of political, diplomatic, economic and*
> *military Domination over the terrorists are the only means to*
> *defeating terrorism.*
> *FOR*
> *the unknown, unfamiliar,*
> *uncomfortable, and arduous pilgrimage*
> *of thinking outside the box by using the knowledge of metaphysics*
> *to bring us toward global healing.*

Enchanted Wisdom

Knowledge of intellect and intelligence is within the realm of logic, reason, rationality and application or interpretation of information. It uses past and present knowledge to plan future action. This can take us to the gateway of wisdom; however, Metaphysics can take us beyond the gateway through expanding our consciousness. There is a process of consciously developing enchanted wisdom. This process has seven components (see figure "*Seven Components of Enchanted Wisdom*"):

Seven Components of Enchanted Wisdom

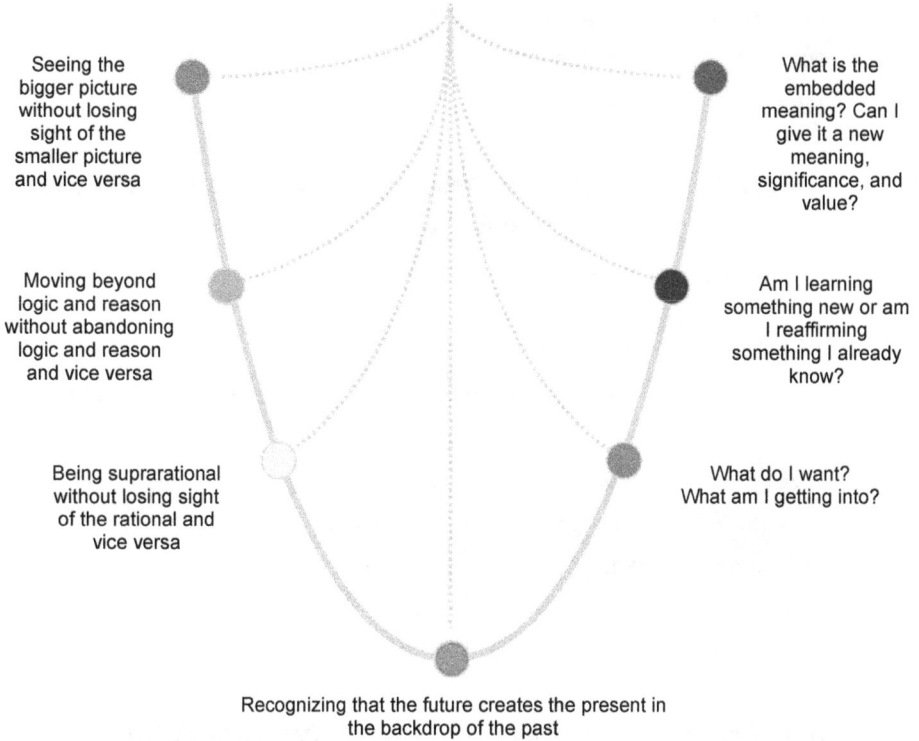

Seeing the bigger picture without losing sight of the smaller picture and vice versa

What is the embedded meaning? Can I give it a new meaning, significance, and value?

Moving beyond logic and reason without abandoning logic and reason and vice versa

Am I learning something new or am I reaffirming something I already know?

Being suprarational without losing sight of the rational and vice versa

What do I want? What am I getting into?

Recognizing that the future creates the present in the backdrop of the past

Future	Present	Past
Where am I going with this action in this pursuit or endeavor?	Where am I now?	Where have I been?

1. **Seeing the bigger picture without losing sight of the smaller picture; likewise, seeing the smaller picture without losing sight of the bigger picture.**

    Looking at the bigger picture in a global perspective, without losing sight of the national political perspective, and looking at national interests without losing sight of global interests.

2. **Moving beyond logic and reason without abandoning them; likewise, using logic and reason without forgetting that something lays beyond them.**

    Logic and reason tells us if we cut off economic sources for terrorist groups and use military force to eliminate them then, we should win.

    However, it is the areas that lack economic stability and security that become the breeding grounds of terrorists because they have nothing to lose and are now given a purpose. Furthermore, hate breeds hate and violence breeds more violence, so we only reinforce their current mindset, allowing it to spread.

    It is time to consider the Metaphysical approach based on the principles of non-violence to win the war on terrorism, rather than taking an eye for an eye and making all of humanity blind. In the 20th century, Mahatma Gandhi achieved this vision of freedom through non-violence nationally. We should focus on taking this to the next level and achieve it globally. Now is the time to consider love, caring and a deeper understanding of each other to avoid Global Suicide.

3. **Being suprarational without losing touch with the rational; likewise, being rational while having the courage to be**

suprarational.

(The Metaphysical definition of suprarational is exceeding the rational by looking beyond rationality for resolutions.)

All dreams and visions begin as suprarational, even though they may appear to be irrational. According to Metaphysics, dreams and visions create possibilities. With conscious pursuit of those dreams and visions, those possibilities become probable. When passionately followed, probabilities become actual and fall from the unbound suprarational into the confines of rational.

Early in the 20th century, Mahatma Gandhi dreamed about winning freedom through the principles of non-violence. He consciously pursued and passionately followed this dream, day in and day out. His dream became reality in 1947. It was a long 40-year journey. The same thing happened with Dr. Martin Luther King when getting the civil rights bill passed, and Nelson Mandela when freeing South Africa from apartheid.

We are in the 21st century, and must dream and envision defeating terrorism with the least possible violence by expanding our consciousness and thinking globally, from nationalism to globalism, from patriotic/nationalistic spirit to global humanistic spirit. Now is the time to take humanity to a new level never seen in human history.

4. **A wise man is always alert and aware of the priorities of the future, present, and past in the following order:**

- **Future – Where am I going in this pursuit or endeavor with these actions, activities, measures, and relationships?**

- Present – Where am I now?
- Past – Where have I been? Where am I coming from and what was the flavor and fashion of my past?

A wise man's awareness is the process of the inclusion of future, present and past.

We need to change the paradigm from our current thinking that the "past creates the present moving towards the future" to the new paradigm "the future creates the present, in the backdrop of the past". Future dreams and visions of Global Healing will take humanity to a new level and will win over terrorism using the Metaphysical principles of resonance. The new resonance will: lift nationalism to globalism and the nationalistic spirit to the global humanistic spirit; create a new resonance for awakening spirituality beyond religions; and create new vistas of hope, bringing about a new Age of Dominion replacing the old Age of Domination.

5. **A wise man always asks himself "Where are my present actions leading me into the future?" This is more critical than the traditional man's "What will it get me?"**

We, humanity at large, should ask our political, military, economic, diplomatic, and religious leaders the question: "Where are our actions, activities, policies and decisions leading humanity in the future? Are they leading us to Global Suicide or do we see light at the end of the tunnel? Do we have to change the direction of our understanding?" Where are our actions leading us globally? We need to move beyond "what will our actions get us nationally?".

6. **A wise man always asks himself "What can I learn that's new?"**

because it is more important than asking "What can I affirm or reaffirm?"

The leaders of Palestine and Israel need to ask the question "Are we learning anything from our past, or are we just affirming and reaffirming that violence breeds violence and hate breeds more hate?" If the leaders do not develop wisdom, then their fighting will go on for many more years. This also applies to India and Pakistan on the Kashmir issue, and now it applies to terrorism in general. There is another way, an elegant way of learning and growing with love, joy and fun in pursuit of spirituality on the path of Metaphysics.

7. **Wisdom is opening new windows to find embedded (traditional) meanings and to create new meanings that have significance. Therefore, a wise man can give value to the newly exposed meanings, which change his feelings and thoughts, and in turn, changes his behavior.**

We, humanity at large, have the ability to find the traditional meanings of politics from the history of mankind, which usually falls under the category of Domination. Domination has now reached its peak and is following the law of diminishing returns of marginal utility. It cannot bring resolution to the current global conflicts. There is nothing more to be gained, but the devastation of humanity. With the passage of time, nuclear and biological technology of weapons of mass destruction will be easily available to many countries and many groups, both terrorists and non-terrorists. One has ten nuclear bombs and the other group has one million nuclear bombs, it makes no difference. Both sides are destructive and have the capability of killing millions of people, where each life is just as precious as the next.

These seven components work together to create the resonance of enchanted wisdom, which will be applied in the following chapters. Now is the time to develop new meaning, significance and value in the form of Dominion. All humanity, including leaders, should listen to their inner wise man. Our leaders are only the trustees of the interests of humanity, not the owners. It is time for humanity to rise to a new level and dawn a new Age of Dominion.

Chapter 5

GLOBAL FAMILY:
HEALING THE ALLIANCE OF NEEDS

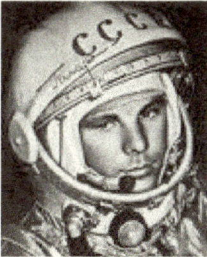

During the cold war period in the 1960's, the first Man in Space, Russian cosmonaut Yuri Gagarin, got a glimpse of the Global Family. When Yuri experienced the vastness of space, he saw the "Blue Planet Earth". Its beauty touched his heart. He said:

"Circling the earth in the orbital spaceship I marveled at the beauty of our planet. People of the world! Let us safeguard and enhance this beauty, not destroy it!"

With large hearts and open minds, we Metaphysically observe humanity as a Global Family looking beyond political, economic and religious boundaries. This is the entire Global Family consisting of grandfathers, grandmothers, fathers, mothers, siblings, cousins, uncles and aunts, nephews and nieces, and people we know and people we do not know, because, we human beings are members of the same family tree. Our roots are so deep that they reach Divinity. We are of the same Divine Energy in different forms. We have chosen to be in this physical universe to experience our journey on this planet. Our Global Family co-exists with the mineral, plant and animal kingdoms. Since we share the planet Earth with other kingdoms, we are all equally responsible for our planet.

Our Global Family consists of many diverse entities at physical, mental, emotional and spiritual levels. At the physical level, the Global Family's differences are color (white, black, brown, red and yellow), gender (male and female), ethnicity, size and shape. At the mental and emotional levels, the Global Family divides itself by intellect (labor, skill and education), by needs (survival, security, belonging and self esteem), and by personality (introvert and extrovert, passive and aggressive, vocal and non-vocal). At the spiritual level, the Global Family separates itself into groups that believe or disbelieve in God (theists and atheists), and those who practice their faith in God through organized religions (Christianity, Islam, Judaism, Hinduism, Buddhism, Jainism, Taoism, Shintoism and many other denominations) or those who explore their own spiritual path.

The guardians of the Global Family, political, economic and religious leaders, are responsible for establishing unity among diversified family members. They are also equally responsible for maintaining co-existence with other kingdoms and the environment to protect our planet. Furthermore, they are responsible for the progress and prosperity of the Global Family by sharing opportunities, knowledge and wealth among the family members with love, caring and compassion. The guardians or leaders of the Global Family should be evaluated and respected according to their contribution to the Global Family and not by how powerful they are. As the old adage states, "with great power comes great responsibility".

94

Let us travel through time and observe humanity's journey from where we started, to where we have come and how we arrived at this crossroad of Global Suicide versus Global Healing.

The expansion of consciousness extends from the early days of primitive man to the present modern civilization and is projected into the future of humanity.

Myriads of souls are separated from Divine Energy, by will, to experience what is beyond Divinity. Similar to a prodigal son who separates from his father, by his will, to experience the world, and then comes back home to his father. This is their journey that started on planet Earth and in the physical universe. In the beginning, primitive man's very survival was challenged by rough weather, and wild animals. After thousands of years, primitive man invented fire to survive in unfriendly environments. "Necessity is the mother of invention", so the necessity for survival invented fire.

After a while, primitive human beings started living together in groups for protection and the population started growing. By living together, they felt secure and dependent upon each other. They developed food to eat, clothing to protect against the weather and huts for living. They satisfied their basic needs of survival and security and started climbing to the next need: that of belonging. They founded neighborhoods and communities.

Some people developed values, and through a sense of esteem they became the leaders. They assumed power and responsibility to make decisions in order to serve and govern their community. These communities evolved into kingdoms and eventually covered the globe. Of great importance was a sense of belonging based on color, race, ethnicity, and political and religious belief systems within differing communities. They developed feelings of competition based on strength, wealth and power, which turned into opposition and then animosity. This animosity led to battles for the expansion of territories, and those who won controlled and manipulated others by imposing their rules, regulations and belief systems on them.

The disparity between the rulers and the people being ruled began to widen and divide people into the haves and have-nots, hopefuls and hopeless, helped and helpless, rational thinkers and fanatics. In the beginning there was apathy among the have-nots, hopeless, and the helpless. When this apathy reached a boiling point, the point beyond tolerance, the downtrodden found new leaders who sympathized with them, and they revolted for independence and freedom. This is what caused the French Revolution, Russian Revolution and Communist Revolution. After these specific revolutions, the victors formed new governments based on ideologies such as socialism and communism.

In other revolutions, people created independence movements and fought for their freedom. They overthrew their rulers and formed new nations including United States of America, Canada, India, and Israel. New governments were formed based on the principles of a republic, giving power back to the people under democratic principles. These governments are by the people, for the people and of the people.

Summarizing the historic evolution of humanity over the last two thousand years, we can say that from years 0 – 1775 A.D., humanity politically evolved through the rulers such as kings, emperors and states, and from 1776 until today, humanity politically evolved through democracy, socialism, communism, dictatorships, military rulers, state rulers and kings.

Through this journey of evolution of the Global Family from primitive man to modern civilization, the following findings are critical for developing resolutions for Global Healing and defeating terrorism:

➤ The Global Family has been evolving on the path of needs. The needs of survival, security, belonging and esteem. At the same time it has been constantly expanding in number and variety. Currently, the Global Family consists of approximately 6 billion diversified people.

➤ Each family member has different needs. Some are merely surviving, some have security issues, and some are part of a community. Survival, security and belonging are basic needs. Very few people grow beyond these basic needs and climb to the next level of need, which is valuing yourself also known as esteem. Those with self esteem become the leaders of various groups, communities, societies and nations.

➤ The leaders govern with a mixed bag of intentions, goals, and missions and can be classified into two major categories. One aims to provide services in congruence with the goals and missions of the groups, communities, societies, nations and United Nations. The other intends to serve their own personal agenda, possibly to gain fame and power, which could have been their motivation to become leaders. Regardless, conflicts are created among the leaders of the various groups, communities, societies and nations. Conflicts turn into skirmishes, which turn into battles, and then into wars among nations on a global level.

➤ Throughout the evolution process, leaders have been using control and manipulation to rule in order to satisfy their personal agendas. In this process the Global Family passes through two major cycles. One cycle is growth and the other is crisis. Crisis creates necessity, and necessity becomes the "mother of invention" for the next growth spurt.

There are two forces that continuously counteracted each other during the historic evolution of the Global Family. One force is the urge to control, rule over and manipulate others, which is the journey of the human ego. The other is the desire for freedom and growth, which is the spiritual journey with the expansion of consciousness. At each evolutionary step, the scale of violence has grown.

Now is the time to expand human consciousness with the path and wisdom of Metaphysics, stretching beyond the knowledge of information, intellect and intelligence so that we can change the paradigm growing with love, joy and fun rather than pain and suffering.

Theory of Needs

There are three major compelling, propelling and driving forces in life. These are human needs, human desires and the human drive to know the mysteries of Life. These forces are interconnected, interdependent and work together integrally and dynamically.

Man's needs are determined by where he is born (space-time location), which family he is born into and what circumstances (political, economical, social and religious) he is passing through. Each human being passes through different stages of needs. For our understanding, let us call them the Hierarchy of Needs as explained in the 20th century by psychologist Abraham Maslow in his theory of needs. According to Maslow, a human being climbs through five rungs of the evolutionary ladder of needs: survival, security, belonging, self-esteem, and self-actualization. The needs of survival, security and belonging are called basic needs.

We are in the 21st century and knowledge has further expanded from information, intellect and intelligence to Metaphysics. Moreover, the needs are extended with the sixth need created by the human drive to know the mysteries of life which is called "knowing". The seventh is the "spiritual need" of developing intimate relationship and partnership with Divine Energy or what we refer to as "God/Goddess/All That Is" (see figure "*Evolutionary Progression of Needs For Coexistence*").

Basic Needs

Let us explore the basic needs of survival, security and belonging and what their roles are in developing vertical gaps and creating divisiveness within the Global Family. Basically human beings live at four levels: physical, mental, emotional and spiritual.

The physical body is the vehicle through which life functions. If there is no physical survival, there is no life. Basically we need good air to breathe, food to eat, water to drink, places to be active, to rest, sleep and to get rid of waste (CO_2, sweat, urine and feces).

Humanity has failed to satisfy the need of survival for all its members, and the gaps between the haves and have-nots, those being helped and the helpless, and the hopeful and hopeless has widened.

> *800 Million People – 13% of mankind – suffer from dire hunger or malnutrition, and 24,000 people die each day from lack of food. Over 1 billion people lack access to clean water and nearly 2 billion lack access to sanitation.*
>
> *However*
>
> *One quarter of the world's population consumes three quarters of the world's oil.*

Evolutionary Progression of Needs for Coexistence

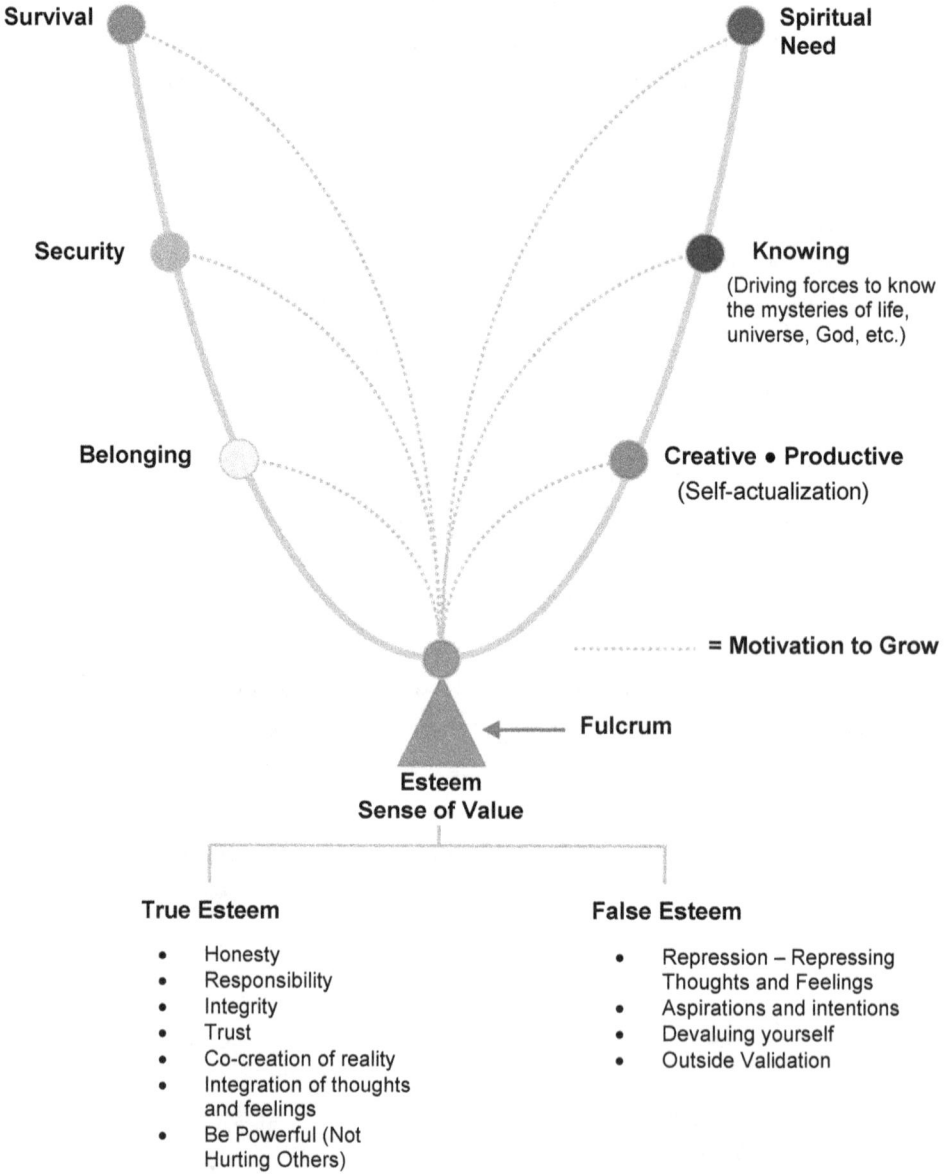

Survival

Spiritual Need

Security

Knowing
(Driving forces to know the mysteries of life, universe, God, etc.)

Belonging

Creative • Productive
(Self-actualization)

············· = Motivation to Grow

← Fulcrum

**Esteem
Sense of Value**

True Esteem

- Honesty
- Responsibility
- Integrity
- Trust
- Co-creation of reality
- Integration of thoughts and feelings
- Be Powerful (Not Hurting Others)

False Esteem

- Repression – Repressing Thoughts and Feelings
- Aspirations and intentions
- Devaluing yourself
- Outside Validation

GLOBAL FAMILY: HEALING THE ALLIANCE OF NEEDS

Security

When the survival needs are taken care of, security needs come next. Human beings become increasingly interested in finding safe places to live, job stability for economic security, physical protection by law and order and stable government for political security.

> *After the 9/11 terrorist acts, the whole world changed. The most secure nation, the United States of America, created a Homeland Security Department. Other developed and underdeveloped countries are still without security, and terrorist acts continue in these nations. The cancer of terrorism has spread throughout the world and has created tremendous fear and anxiety. This has increased the gap between people being helped by security and those who are helpless because they have no security.*

Belonging

After satisfying the basic need of security, human beings can focus on their need of belonging with other people and society. In our daily life, this is exhibited as the need and desire to marry, have a family and be a part of a community. We want to affiliate with service, labor and professional organizations, be members of political parties, members of religious organizations, brothers in fraternities, sisters in sororities or a part of a gang or Jihad group. Human beings are susceptible to loneliness and anxieties, and belonging is a natural instinct and antidote.

The need to belong, has created many diverse groups physically, mentally and emotionally in political parties, economic strata, races, ethnic groups, ideologies, and religions. Diversities are beautiful if they are balanced and harmonious, but when they are out of balance, diversity turns into divisions that cause conflicts. If the conflicts are not resolved constructively then they turn into battles, which in turn lead to war.

One conflict that repeatedly occurs at the physical level is due to gender. For centuries, men have dominated societies. Since the industrial revolution, women have fought for equal rights and liberation. The resulting conflicts can be easily resolved for betterment of society because men need women and women need men. They complement and supplement each other. If we maintain this progress toward the emancipation of women, women will be equally respected in the 21st century in all phases of life.

Another conflict that occurs at the physical level is due to skin color or race. Constant conflicts between the races are caused because of the claim that one race has superiority over another.

> *Over history the whites took land from the American Indians and enslaved blacks. Conflicts between white people and the American Indians were resolved by giving them back some of their own land. Conflicts between whites and blacks resulted in the civil rights movement started under the leadership of Martin Luther King, who espoused the principles of non-violence, eventually leading to the Civil Rights Act, which was passed during the Kennedy/Johnson Administration. Discrimination has diminished, but has a long way to go.*

Any conflict arising at the physical level can be easily diagnosed and resolved through movements of non-violence, dialogues, negotiations, and civil rights bills.

The mental and emotional sense of belonging has created several divisions. The first major division is created by geopolitical boundaries, commonly known as nationalism – "I am American. I am Canadian. I am French. I am Indian. I am Japanese. I am Chinese. I am Israeli…"

The second major set of differences is at the economic and ideological levels: rich, middle class and poor; white collar and blue collar; capitalist, socialist and communist; and the haves and have-nots. The vertical gap between haves and have-nots is constantly expanding as discussed previously.

> *Since the Second World War there have been constant conflicts, which are at times resolved by various organizations through dialogue, negotiation, treaties and international trade. The major ideological conflict between Communism and the free world created the cold war period, where there was a massive build-up of weapons of mass destruction after the Second World War. The fall of the Berlin Wall and the collapse of the USSR in the late 1980s became a turning point for humanity from Global Suicide to Global Healing.*

The third major set of conflicts is created at the mental, emotional and spiritual levels. There are numerous diverse religions in the Global Family. Every human being has a relationship with a Divine Energy, generally known as God. Whether he or she believes in God (theist) or not (atheist), there is still a relationship. This relationship is called spirituality. Religion is the pathway to the establishment of this relationship with God. According to the general public, religion is a specific system of belief, with rules and rituals. There have been various belief systems established throughout centuries, which turned into institutions and became organized religions.

The majority of humanity hold onto their religious beliefs firmly as they have been deeply rooted in their subconscious mind since childhood. These religious beliefs and attitudes are part of their life script and have created major conflicts throughout history of mankind turning into violence, killing, pain and suffering.

Currently, we are passing through conflicts of religious beliefs resulting in the war on terrorism. This has widened the vertical gap between the fanatics and the rational thinkers. Fanatics cover up what they don't know by imposing their beliefs on others. They believe they are right and you are wrong unless you accept their belief. Rational thinkers say you may be right, you may be wrong or we both may be right, so let us have a dialogue and share our knowledge, combine it with logic and reason and develop rationale for this belief.

Humanity has to seek new knowledge with innovative approaches to resolve these conflicts. These are further explored in the next two books, *GLOBAL HEALING: Awakening Spirituality* and *GLOBAL HEALING: New Vistas of Hope.*

Self Esteem

The leaders are climbers, climbing to the fourth need of self-esteem. They make the choices and decisions and create reality for the Global Family. Therefore, it is critical to understand the mindset of the leaders. Let us explore how those leaders have brought us to this crossroad of war on terrorism leading towards Global Suicide and how we can change to the pathway toward Global Healing by using Metaphysical enchanted wisdom.

Since the incidents of 9/11, the Global Family has been distressed. The source of distress personally, nationally and globally is coming from two major elements. One is fear created by terrorism and the other is low self-esteem because of feeling insecure. We are in a downward spiral: fear breeds fear; hate produces hate and violence incites violence. Freedom is in jeopardy. Somehow, we have to stop this downward spiral and turn around. These two elements or issues are so profound and so powerful that the havoc they reap is immense. So, while the Global

Family has declared the war on terrorism, we are passing through low self-esteem at the same time.

The need for self-esteem is an elusive concept compared to the basic needs of survival, security and belonging. Esteem is a value judgment. In the modern age, judgments are considered bad, as the bible says "Judge ye not, lest you be judged." There is a great difference between being judgmental and having value judgments. Value judgments are the hierarchy of priorities.

Esteem is elusive because evaluations are often emotional and subject to change. Every emotion, from the most frivolous to the most sincere, from the meaningless to the most powerful, is a reflection of self-esteem and is produced out of self-esteem. Every thought is also motivated through and a product of self-esteem. Therefore, self-esteem can be elusive because it is emotionally involved and subjective.

Within the hierarchy of needs, self-esteem is the fourth priority. Although it is the fourth priority, in order to have self-esteem, you must have already filled the needs of survival, security and belonging.

The reason that self-esteem is so elusive is because even though we are completely surrounded by self-esteem issues, we never really experience self-esteem as whole. Just as a fish does not understand the water it is swimming within, we do not understand self-esteem, yet we are completely immersed in self-esteem. Every emotion we have, every thought we have, every action that we take involves our self-esteem.

Why is self-esteem so important? Because life is about growing, learning, having fun, consciously creating success, exploring, encountering, and self-reflecting. Whatever you are doing in this life, it involves growth. In order for growth to occur, we need motivation. We need a reason to stretch, to reach, to explore, and to understand. Esteem provides this motivation and the reason to grow.

Esteem is our self-estimation of ourselves. Our esteem is what motivates us to make new choices and new beliefs that bring about change. It is esteem that gives us the will to explore change and to see the paradigm of thinking in new ways at a higher level. Our current methods of winning the war on terrorism are created based on the knowledge of information, intellect and intelligence and they are not sufficient. Therefore, we have to begin thinking at the Metaphysical level.

Our capacity of survival is predicated by our ability to think and feel, and to do something with those thoughts and feelings. Our ability to reason, is to take thoughts and feelings and organize them in such a way that they create something that is more impactful than either thought or feeling alone. In order to think and feel productively, it is important to measure our impact, to see clearly through self-appraisal and to have a sense of value. Esteem provides that measure, that motivation, that value.

Esteem is critical because every power that we have as human beings is predicated by our self-evaluation, our estimate of who we are. Our willingness and ability to act comes out of our self-esteem. If we do not have self-esteem we will shrink into the shadow of existence, relinquish our power and render ourselves impotent. Without self-esteem, we would not survive. Now is the time to raise our self-esteem back to the levels when we first put the man on the moon and all of humanity watched and celebrated in unison around the globe. Now is the time to grow and to change our reality by making new choices that turn into new beliefs that will shift our path from Global Suicide to Global Healing.

Self-esteem is essential not just to sustaining life. It is essential for existence. To elaborate further, esteem is the evaluation and estimate of values that we make for ourselves and adhere to. Esteem is the love we earn, upon which we evaluate, estimate and appraise ourselves, our worth, our value and our right to exist.

Therefore, it is important to differentiate between true-esteem and false-esteem. All leaders of humanity develop self-esteem. The constructive and creative leaders in the 20th century have true-esteem, such as Mahatma Gandhi, Martin Luther King, and Nelson Mandela. Destructive and constraining leaders have false-esteem, such as Mussolini, Hitler, Stalin, Saddam Hussein and Bin Laden. The destiny of humanity is directed and guided by a few political, economic, social and religious leaders. So, it is very important to seek true esteem as opposed to false esteem.

What is true esteem? True esteem has seven major components: honesty; responsibility; integrity; trust; co-creation; integration of thoughts and feelings; and a sense of power without hurting others. These seven components work together to create synergy of true esteem.

True esteem is based on being honest with yourself, and honest in your determination to be willing and responsible for a situation no matter how bad it becomes. It is based on responsibility to yourself and others. How willing are you to take responsibility? How quickly, how elegantly? The answers to those questions trigger your ability to think faster, think creatively, focus and feel emotions more deeply, more profoundly, and more intensely through a wide range - from passion to compassion. With regard to the integration of thoughts and feelings, how much do you honor your emotions? How much do you let yourself listen to your feelings, understand what you are feeling, and use it as feedback without letting it run your life? True esteem also involves integrity, which relates to the character of the person, and trust. How much do you trust yourself? Are you trustworthy? When you trust yourself, you are willing to understand yourself. This in turn creates seeking, understanding and meaning with more perception and conception.

How much effort do you put into co-creating with your partners and coworkers in the physical world and the Divine Energy in the Metaphysical world? Willingness to co-create generates humility and enhances character. Finally true esteem makes you aware that you are not helpless. You can ask for help. You can do things for yourself. You can work for yourself and with others. You are not helpless.

Those that seek esteem without including the above components establish false esteem. What is false esteem? False esteem is created by repressing your thoughts and feelings and by making choices out of fear. It is motivating yourself out of fear, rather than out of growth, doing things not because you want to do them, but you are afraid not to. For example: Do you help an old lady cross the street, for fear of what people may think of you if you didn't, or do you do it because you genuinely feel an inner drive to unselfishly help a fellow human in their time of need?

False esteem comes from your capacity to cynically devalue your resources. Everything that is going to happen is going to happen. Much of the whole doom and gloom scenario pronouncing the final warning, day of reckoning, judgment day, is based on the fact that we have no choice anymore. You feel the decisions you make don't matter anyway.

People also seek false esteem through aspiration and intention. You intend to do something in the future, but you want the credit now. Similarly, you aspire to be this or that person therefore you want the special privileges that may come with that future person. Living on intention and aspiration is frequently a source of false esteem. Generally, political campaigns in democratic countries are run based on the aspiration and intention to do something in the future.

The most common way of getting false esteem is wanting outside validation. Seeking outside valuation as a form of self-esteem is devastating. There is nothing wrong with outside validation. Everybody needs it but it should not be used as a source of self-esteem. Instead, it should be used as a source of feedback, income, or validation. When outside validation becomes a source of self-esteem, it becomes false esteem and it will create havoc. In the history of mankind, maximum havoc was created by the leaders who have sought outside validation as a source of esteem, leaders such as Mussolini, Hitler, Stalin, Saddam Hussein and Bin Laden. The political, economic, religious and social leaders who have sought outside validation as a source of self-esteem, have contributed more to the conflicts than to finding its resolutions. They are the ones that have brought the Global Family closer and closer to Global Suicide.

After 9/11, humanity's self-esteem dropped like a lead balloon. People were seized by fear all over America and throughout the world. Self-esteem became imprisoned by doubt, worry and confusion. People suppressed their own thoughts and feelings and began to make choices based on fear. The government grounded all planes, and people stored multiple days of food and remained inside their homes. The political, financial, religious and social leaders lifted their intentions of doing something about terrorism with more of an eye on outside validation than on doing the right thing. Relatives of the casualties of the twin towers became totally powerless and miserable. All of America passed through great depression and anger. People became bitter, resentful and cynical. They became physically, mentally and emotionally drained and were obsessed with the news on television. Leaders competed with each other in the expression of their intentions, aspirations, plans, ideas, and executions.

Self-Actualization

After satisfying the basic needs of survival, security, belonging and self-esteem, a few human beings are able to climb to the fifth need of self-actualization. In the self-esteem need, the motivating forces are value judgments, estimates, evaluations and appraisals of themselves. When human beings earn that self-esteem, they want to grow further. Some engage this motivation to grow and realize that they have the ability to create, develop and to produce something new. They evolve a continuous desire to fulfill the potential "to be all that they can be". It is a matter of becoming the most complete person possible, which is called self-actualization.

To be truly self-actualized, you need to have your basic needs filled, at least to a considerable extent. When your basic needs are unmet you cannot fully devote yourself to fulfilling your potential. Therefore, only a very small percentage of the world's population is truly self-actualized. Who are the self-actualized people? If you go through recent history, we come across several self-actualizing personalities. In the political arena Thomas Jefferson, Abraham Lincoln, Mahatma Gandhi, Martin Luther King and Nelson Mandela come to mind. In science and technology, Thomas Edison, Benjamin Franklin, Albert Einstein are leading candidates. In literature Khalil Gibran, William Wardsworth, Rabindranath Tagore, Robert Frost, Mark Twain and Ralph Waldo Emmerson are at the top of the list. They could differentiate between true and false, honest and dishonest and the fake and genuine. Their hearts responded to the soul's call to adventure with goodness when there was injustice, discrimination, misery or violence. They appreciated beauty on all levels - physical, mental, emotional and spiritual.

110

Knowing

The purpose of human life is to grow and growth is driven by three types of forces. One is the *compelling* force to satisfy needs. The ultimate need in human life is spirituality, to love and to be loved, to be loving and being loving. The second is the *propelling* force to satisfy your desires. The ultimate desire is to be happy and joyful. The third is the *driving* force to know the mysteries of life. Why do I exist? What am I and what is the purpose of life? Where am I coming from and where am I going? What is this universe made of and how is it being operated? There is no end to knowing (see figure "*Forces of Human Growth*").

Knowing goes beyond knowledge. Knowledge is the accumulation of information, interpretation by intellect, and synthesis by intelligence. Knowledge is within the realm of logic, reason and rationality. Knowing is the dynamism of understanding. It is experiencing the understanding.

> One morning, Aristotle was walking on the beach of the Mediterranean Sea. He saw an old man digging a hole in the sand with a small bucket at his side. Aristotle observed him and walked away. The next morning he saw the same old man, digging a bigger hole in the sand with a bigger bucket next to him. Aristotle wondered what the old man was doing.

> A week later, he was walking on the same beach. There was the same old man, filling the hole with a bucket full of water. Aristotle was curious and he stopped to watch him again. The man did the same thing over and over. He went to the sea, filled the bucket with water, went back to the hole and emptied the bucket of water into the hole.

> Aristotle approached the old man and asked the question: "What are you doing my friend?" The old man answered: "Don't you

111

Forces of Human Growth

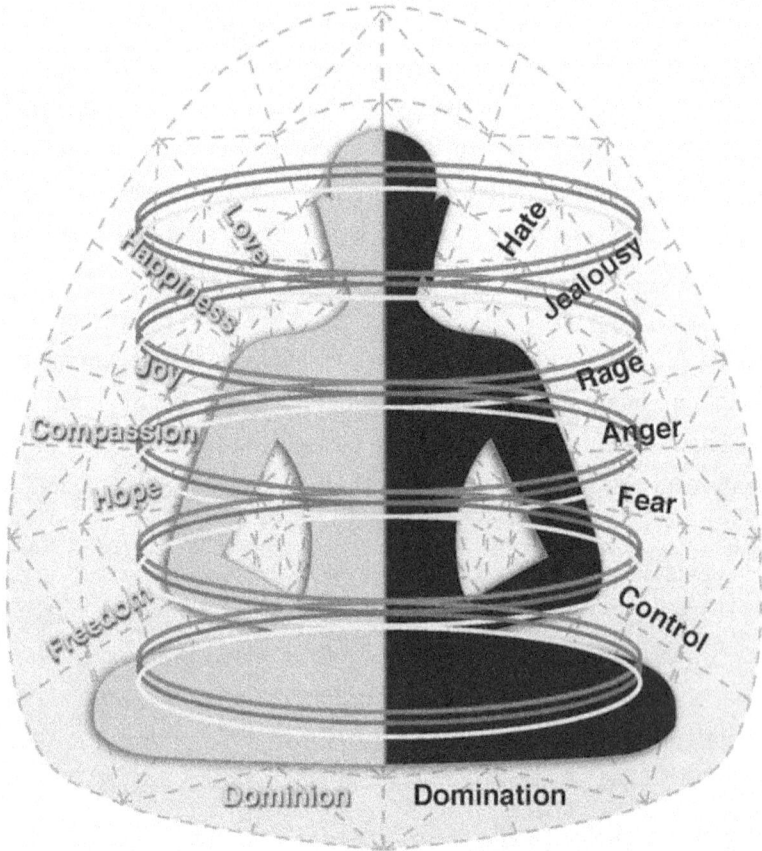

Compelling Force of Needs from Survival to the Ultimate Need of Love.

Propelling Force of Desire from Satisfying Needs to the Ultimate Desire of Being Happy and Joyful.

Driving Force of Knowing from Accomplishing Desires to the Ultimate Drive of Knowing the Mysteries of Life

112

see me? I am trying to empty the sea." Aristotle started laughing. "How can you empty a sea by filling a small hole with buckets of water?" The old man threw the bucket and burst into laughter. Aristotle didn't understand why the old man was laughing, so he asked him and the old man said, "you are probably right, but let me ask you, how can you empty the mysteries of life with your small bucket of logic and reason?" and then walked away. Aristotle later discovered the old man was the mystic Heraclitus, also known as Heraclitus the Obscure, Heraclitus the Dark, Heraclitus the Riddling.

The knowledge of information, intellect and intelligence can only identify with what, when, where, how and why something happens and they cannot go beyond that. Knowing is the ability to know the root cause of emotions such as hate and anger, and the ability to provide solutions along with means. Mahatma Gandhi did this in the 20th century at the national level, why can't we do it at a global level? Knowing takes you beyond the paradoxes and opens the door of wisdom. Metaphysically, the driving force of knowing takes you to the gateway of spirituality.

Spiritual Need

Spirituality is a relationship between an individual and the Divine Energy often referred to as God or in its more fuller sense, God/Goddess/All That Is. The progression of spiritual need grows from curiosity, to knowledge, to seeking and then to devotion. In an individual's life, the spiritual need starts with curiosity to know God, and know about God, by attending traditional places of worship. The thirst for spirituality grows by acquiring knowledge about God through reading scriptures, spiritual and philosophical books and taking religious or spiritual classes.

The majority of the members of the Global Family are only curious because they are too busy satisfying their basic needs. A small group of members of the Global Family become knowledgeable persons or scholars such as priests, rabbis, gurus, mullahs, pundits, teachers and professors of philosophy and theology.

Out of those scholars, very few go on to realize that informative, intellectual and intelligent knowledge of God is borrowed knowledge. This knowledge may be true or false, but it is not personal experience. They want to personally experience Divinity so they turn into seekers. In the modern age the seekers are called Metaphysicians. With total dedication, the Metaphysicians turn into mapmakers, making spiritual maps for themselves and for the rest of the Global Family.

Lifting Self-Esteem by Healing
Metaphysically:

> *We, the members of the Global Family, create our own reality, and*
> *we are responsible for what we are.*
> *We are the masters of our destiny, and*
> *not the victims of fate.*

We, the members of the Global Family, have created the war on terrorism leading towards Global Suicide. We gave the power to our political, economic and religious leaders who have been making choices and decisions on our behalf and have brought us to this junction. We, the members of the Global Family and our leaders, have to work together and embrace Metaphysical wisdom to create Global Healing.

What do we want? What are we getting into? We want to have peace so we can work together, progress and prosper as one loving and caring family, standing tall among all intelligences in the physical universe. So why are we bringing ourselves closer to suicide?

114

Are we learning something new or are we reaffirming what we have done in the past? We have been using political, military, diplomatic, religious approaches, United Nation resolutions, cease fires and treaties for the last 100 years. They have put us in two periods, one is preparation for war and the other is war itself. Each successive war is on a larger scale. We are just reaffirming the same patterns again and again.

We need to find the embedded and historical meaning of our methodology, which causes the same cycle of preparation of war and actual war. We then need to create new visions that promote Global Healing.

Usually what is written in history are the highlights of actions taken by political, economical, military and religious leaders including their hidden personal agendas of name, fame, power and glory. Metaphysical wisdom seeks new meaning, significance and value of Dominion, which includes cooperation, coexistence and co-creation.

According to Metaphysical wisdom, the focal point is the fulcrum of self-esteem. Currently we are experiencing an imbalanced shift in that fulcrum due to fear, which has led to the building of armed war camps. This imbalance has converted the diversity of family members into divisions. Healing of the alliance of needs is crucial, especially after 9/11, to lift the self-esteem of the entire Global Family. Metaphysically, healing can be done by shifting the fulcrum of self-esteem back into balance in four steps (see figure *"Healing the Alliance of Needs By Shifting the Position of the Fulcrum of Self-Esteem"*).

The first step in generating true self-esteem is to recognize and realize we create our own reality and we are responsible for what we created on 9/11. We must acknowledge and accept the responsibility that this is our creation. At the same time, we must learn why we caused it so it will not

Healing the Alliance of Needs
By Shifting Position of the Fulcrum of Self-Esteem

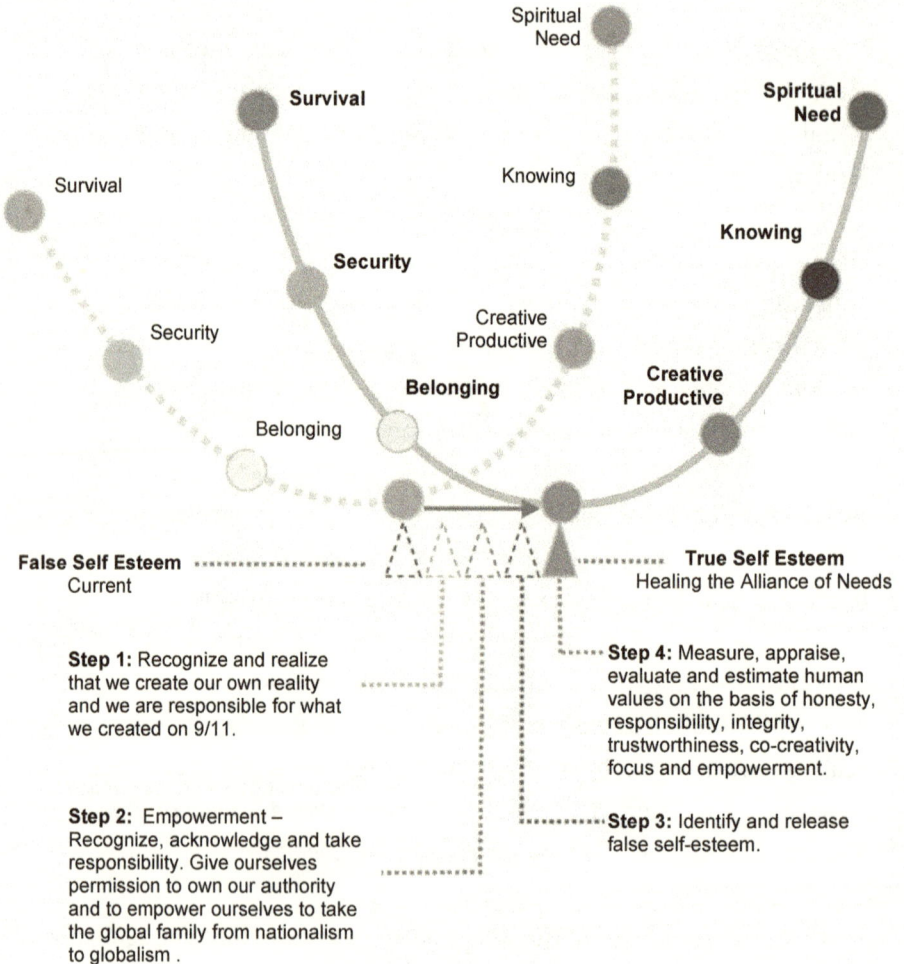

Spiritual Need

Survival

Spiritual Need

Survival

Knowing

Knowing

Security

Creative Productive

Security

Creative Productive

Belonging

Belonging

Belonging

False Self Esteem
Current

True Self Esteem
Healing the Alliance of Needs

Step 1: Recognize and realize that we create our own reality and we are responsible for what we created on 9/11.

Step 4: Measure, appraise, evaluate and estimate human values on the basis of honesty, responsibility, integrity, trustworthiness, co-creativity, focus and empowerment.

Step 2: Empowerment – Recognize, acknowledge and take responsibility. Give ourselves permission to own our authority and to empower ourselves to take the global family from nationalism to globalism .

Step 3: Identify and release false self-esteem.

116

be repeated. Only through responsibility can we lift our self-esteem.

The second step is to give ourselves permission to empower ourselves to take the Global Family to a new level from nationalism to globalism and patriotism to humanism to win the war on terrorism.

The third step is to identify and turn away from false esteem.

> *We, the members of the Global Family, have to develop courage to confront our fears. We need to abandon choices based on fear by releasing our repressed thoughts and feelings. We have to be innovative, imaginative and inventive in making choices and decisions to win the war on terrorism with the least possible violence and killing, changing the mindsets of terrorists. We have to expand our consciousness and awaken spirituality to inspire the Global Family to see that better days are ahead because we are masters of our own destinies, not victims of fate. We have to select and elect leaders who are genuine in their intentions and aspirations and will use Metaphysical wisdom in creating their dreams and visions. We will have leaders who can think "outside the box" making new choices and decisions rather than continuing to lead based on traditional thinking. The dreams and visions should be for the Global Family in congruence with the national family. We must awaken the Global Family to support leaders who have genuine intention rather than those who are looking for outside validation from the general public.*

The fourth step is to measure, appraise, evaluate and estimate human values on the basis of honesty and responsibility; of integrity and trustworthiness; and of co-creativity focused with empowerment.

117

These are the steps for humanity to shift the fulcrum of self-esteem, which in turn will lift the self-esteem of the Global Family. They will have a heightened feeling of love, trust, expectancy and enthusiasm. The Global Family will be full of creativity with innovative ideas, imagination and inventions. The Global Family will take pride in accomplishing the awakening of consciousness in the 21st century just as we are proud of the progress of science and technology in the 20th century. The Global Family will be more courageous to venture into new realms taking us from the old Age of Domination to the new Age of Dominion.

Chapter 6

THE WAYS OF METAPHYSICS: PORTALS TO THE FUTURE

The ways of Metaphysics are:
  Individually:

I create my own reality, and
I am responsible for what I am.

  Collectively:

We, the members of the Global Family, create our own reality, and
we are responsible for what we are.

There is a familiar saying, "God helps those who help themselves". Similarly, the ways of Metaphysics are born out of a sense of responsibility. Metaphysically, the secret of responsibility is:

The more responsibility we take, the more secrets of Global Healing will be revealed to us.

The more we blame each other, the secrets we know about Global Healing will be taken away from us.

121

Responsibility is not a simple reaction. According to the Webster Dictionary, the meaning of responsibility is: "The condition, quality, fact or instance of being responsible, answerable, accountable, or liable, for a person, family, trust or office". The meaning of reaction is: "a return or opposing action or influence; a response as to a stimulus or influence." Human reaction, individually or collectively, to any incident is stimulated by the subconscious mind, and it is usually impulsive.

> *A Palestinian suicide bomber killed twenty children on a school bus and injured fifty by-standers in Jerusalem. The immediate response from the Israeli government was retaliation using air missiles to kill Hamas leaders in the Gaza Strip. The Palestinians impulsively responded with another suicide bomb. These responses are reactive rather than responsible. These violent reactions have continued for more than fifty years without any resolution. These reactions repeat a vicious cycle spiraling downward, causing terrorism to spread throughout the world. We, the members of the Global Family, have either caused it by actual participation politically, economically, militarily or religiously, or we have allowed it to happen.*

Responsibility is the key for human growth, progress and prosperity. So we, the members of the Global Family, are responsible for what we are and the dangerous world we live in, a world with terrorism. We need to inquire and investigate how we created this dangerous world, how we caused it so we can change the direction.

As previously explored, more than 90% of the members of the Global Family are relatively busy satisfying their own basic needs of survival, security and belonging. Therefore, they give their responsibility to the guardians of the Global Family who are either the elected leaders, kings, dictators or military rulers. Included in the mix are the leaders of organized religions, who assume the responsibility for religious beliefs and systems. All these leaders are in the fourth stage of need, the self-esteem need. They take the responsibility for leadership and make choices and decisions on behalf of their people. During the second world war, when the atom bombs killed millions of people in Hiroshima and Nagasaki, the members of the Global Family were shocked and realized through pain and suffering that this is not the way that we should live. Pressure mounted on the leaders and the United Nations was formed to resolve conflicts among the nations without going through wars. This was a difficult way to learn a lesson. In spite of all the lessons we learned in the first and second world wars, and passing through the cold war period, we are now here and living in a dangerous world of terrorism. Let us explore where we have gone wrong through the use of the Metaphysical components of wisdom.

The guardians of the Global Family have a responsibility to establish a balance and harmony among the widely diverse family members. Balance and harmony can only be established if the leaders follow the laws of cooperation and co-creation by working together. However, they are competitive, lured by the false-esteem of outside validation. Thus, they have created divisions among the Global Family, creating rivalry and animosity, which ultimately turns into hate, anger, revenge and violence. These leaders have the constrictive consciousness of thinking "inside the box". They have been making choices and decisions based on their own interests in personal status, control, power to rule over others and manipulation. Thus, they have created the present war on terrorism.

In reality, we the members of the Global Family, also have created the present reality of hostility and terrorism by allowing our leaders to make choices and decisions on our behalf. So we are equally responsible for everything happening today. There are seven components of constrictive consciousness of thinking "inside the box" that are creating the present reality of the war on terrorism (see figure "*Constrictive Consciousness of Thinking Inside The Box*").

The first component of constrictive consciousness is focusing on minute details while losing sight of the bigger picture, and focusing on large ideological concepts while losing sight of the smaller concrete issues.

> *Most political national leaders see the smaller picture of nationalism and patriotism while losing sight of globalism and humanism. The United Nations and the super powers are the only political organizations that have taken responsibility for the bigger picture of globalism and humanism without losing sight of the smaller picture of the national interests of fellow members. These organizations have made great progress since World War II, but it has not been enough to establish globalism and humanism.*

> *The recent war on Iraq was not about what happened on 9/11, instead it was about changing the regime in Iraq, which resulted in a loss of unity among the member-states within the United Nations. All political leaders talk about global peace, the roadmap to peace in the Middle East and establishing democracy in Iraq, but we have ended up with an expansion of hostilities. It appears that we lack the wisdom of cooperation and co-creation.*

> *Similarly, religious leaders see the smaller picture of their own organized religions, and focus on their doctrines and dogmas without trying to understand that we are members of the same Global Family and the children of the same Divinity. They also talk about global peace and compassion, loving and caring for each other and create interfaith/religious organizations,*

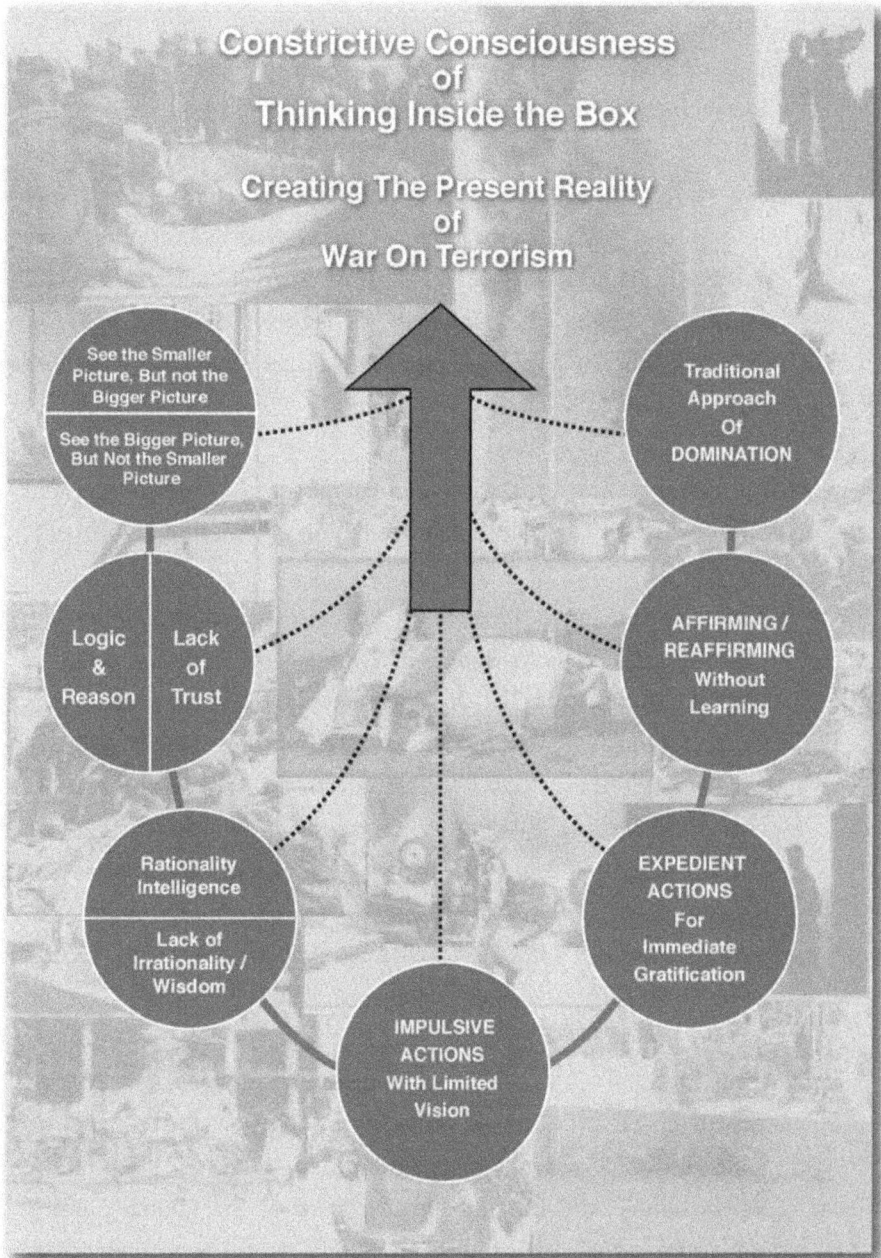

Constrictive Consciousness
of
Thinking Inside the Box

Creating The Present Reality
of
War On Terrorism

See the Smaller Picture, But not the Bigger Picture

See the Bigger Picture, But Not the Smaller Picture

Traditional Approach Of DOMINATION

Logic & Reason

Lack of Trust

AFFIRMING / REAFFIRMING Without Learning

Rationality Intelligence

Lack of Irrationality / Wisdom

EXPEDIENT ACTIONS For Immediate Gratification

IMPULSIVE ACTIONS With Limited Vision

conferences and seminars for understanding each other's faiths. People lose sight of the fact that their organizations and their leaders have their own personal agendas of control, power over and manipulation of their followers.

The religious rift has become so deep that there are people willing to die in the name of their God in order to kill any others that do not agree with their religious beliefs. The maximum amount of killing and violence has happened in the name of religions that are supposed to spread the message of loving and caring for humanity.

The second component of constrictive consciousness is using logic and reason while forgetting something that lies beyond them, namely trust.

While dealing with the natural world it is essential to probe, question and to understand matter and the physical laws of Mother Nature. In the 20th century, the Global Family was totally focused on the development of science and technology. In fact, the whole education system is based on logic and reason. Therefore, individually and collectively, the mindset of the 20th century human is ingrained with logic, reason, and open-ended inquiry. However, when it comes to the human emotions, religious beliefs, attitudes and relationships, logic and reason cannot establish balance and harmony.

Many leaders forget about trust. Trust can heal relationships and generate the synergy of co-creation. Trust starts with self trust and expands to trusting your family members, your neighbors, trusting your community, trusting your country and trusting the members of the Global Family. All current approaches consisting of negotiations, treaties, and cease-fires have a legal basis but they are implemented too often without trust.

Religious leaders talk about trust, compassion and love. They tell many stories and anecdotes from the scriptures but do not share the procedures of how to develop trust.

The third component of constrictive consciousness is:
Being rational without having the courage to be suprarational*
OR
Being suprarational while losing touch with rationality.
 * The Metaphysical definition of suprarational is "beyond rational"

According to the Webster Dictionary the meaning of the word rational is: "based on or derived from reasoning; able to reason; showing reason; not foolish or silly; the fundamental reason or rational basis of something; a statement, exposition of explanation of reasons or principles."

Rationality follows logic and reason. As discussed previously, logic, reason and rationality have progressed exponentially in the 20th century because of the development of science and technology. The whole education system is based on a rational thinking process. All political, military and financial leaders, with few exceptions, are basically rational beings. The use of logic, reason and rationality have done wonders in exploring the physical sciences and developing technology. However, when dealing with human relationships, logic, reason and rationality have their limitations, especially when dealing with fanatic mindsets. Infact, they have been counterproductive and have brought us to the crossroad of Global Suicide versus Global Healing. All the leaders that make choices and decisions on the behalf of members of the Global Family are basically rational thinkers, who think "inside the box" and do not have the courage to be supra-rational (beyond rational), to dream. The great leaders in the history of the Global Family, those who changed the direction from destruction to progression, were dreamers, but they never lost touch with rationality. They were practical and pragmatic.

When you turn on the television and surf the channels you see the same message using rationality but with different words. For example: The news says that there is a big explosion at the U.N. office in Iraq; twenty-five people die and one hundred people are injured. The focus of the report is on: Who did it? How did they do it? Why did they do it? Who is taking responsibility for it? Whom do we blame? It centers on the facts of what happened. Thus, the whole consciousness has been constricted to the immediate concrete level rather than expanding consciousness to find the root cause of the terrorist act, which lies in hate and anger. If we cure the hate and anger, then we cure terrorism. It is as if the branches are being cut off the tree of terrorism, rather than removing the roots of hate and anger.

Each country has created a special agency or department such as the U.S. Central Intelligence Agency. These agencies can find incidents of conflicts and terrorism, but cannot resolve the issues causing them. We have to look beyond intelligence and create a special department, The Central Wisdom Agency (CWA) of the 21st century, to bring resolution to conflicts and win the war on terrorism.

The fourth component of constrictive consciousness involves impulsive actions taken with limited vision of the future consequences.

The attack on Iraq, which was against the wishes of the United Nations, lacked a comprehensive exit plan. These actions lacked any consideration of the future relationship with members of the United Nations and set the dangerous and short-sighted precedent of aggression first.

The fifth component of constrictive consciousness has more focus on immediate gratification. 'What will it get us now?' rather than 'Where are my actions leading us (in the future)?'

Political leaders are motivated by either true or false self-esteem. False esteem is based on repression and fear, false aspirations and intentions and outside validation. The leaders who are motivated by false esteem repress the population stressing fearful consequences (acts of terror) so they can maintain poll ratings in democratic countries. They are more focused on what they will get now rather than where this will lead to in the future. They take expedient actions for immediate gratification. Leaders who are motivated by true esteem are honest, responsible, have integrity, trustworthiness and foresight for co-creation.

The political evolution of democracy over the last two hundred years has expanded the active participation of people in election of their leaders and policy and decision making processes. According to the bell curve, 80% of the population has an average knowledge base and I.Q. Leaders who speak the language of the average people win elections. Therefore, policies and decisions of these leaders tend to lack vision. The evolutionary process of democracy will lead to the next level - meritocracy. Meritocracy will lift the bar for voter qualifications. In meritocracy, a person should be qualified to vote at the age of eighteen only after completing certain basic courses in political science, world history, civics and psychology, similar to the process of getting a driver's license. This will in turn lift the quality of the leaders who will make principle-based actions rather than expedient reactions.

129

The sixth component of constrictive consciousness is more focused on affirming and reaffirming the past, rather than learning for the future.

> *Are we learning anything, or just affirming and reaffirming the past using more advanced weaponry?*

> *The Palestinians and Israelis have been continually preparing for and fighting war. These wars are under the name of religion, fighting for the holy land. Every time we affirm and reaffirm our policies under the name of religion we create more and more violence on a larger scale, causing a downward spiraling cycle. The answer to breaking this cycle can be found in the way of Metaphysics.*

The seventh component of constrictive consciousness uses the traditional approach of Domination supported by the collective unconscious. There is a lack of courage to think "outside the box", and go beyond the mass psychology of Domination.

The Webster Dictionary meaning of the word Domination is, "to rule; to govern; to control; to predominate over." The Global Family has been living in the Age of Domination throughout history of mankind. As the Global Family has been evolving from barbarianism to modern civilization, the forms of Domination have been evolving from barbaric ruling to the current modern sophisticated and complex form of Domination. Since the 18th century, the Global Family has been slowly moving toward democracy or government by the people, for the people and of the people.

Along with the evolution of the Global Family, the power to rule, to govern, and control has shifted from warriors to political parties, to organized religions, to laborers/proletariats and to business entrepreneurs.

The current Age of Domination is very complex and intricate. Metaphysically, it consists of control; power to rule over others; manipulation; reliving the past; an unfriendly world; to take or be taken; and to blame or be blamed. All these components are interacting and interwoven with each other creating complexity (see figure *"Current Age of Domination"*).

The first component of Domination is control. Control comes out of insecurity and it is the opposite of freedom. Freedom is a vital prerequisite for political, religious and economic growth. So there are constant battles and trade offs between control and freedom. Right now, the growth of the Global Family is going at a snail's pace along a pathway of pain and suffering.

Politically, democracy was established on the principle of freedom and government elected by the people. Freedom is gaining more ground over control, and the growth of the Global Family has accelerated. The members of the Global Family joined together to work for freedom, and the United Nations was formed. People began to understand their right to freedom, slavery has diminished, discrimination is reduced, women are getting equal rights, but still we are in the Age of Domination.

With regard to religion, we are making progress toward freedom to choose a faith to practice. Some members of the Global Family have come to respect and understand differing religious beliefs. Some are developing the capacity to take the best out of every religious belief system and creating the new age of spirituality beyond religion. However, too many members of the Global Family are psychologically controlled by their religious beliefs and some of them become fanatics. The gap between the rational thinkers and fanatics has increased

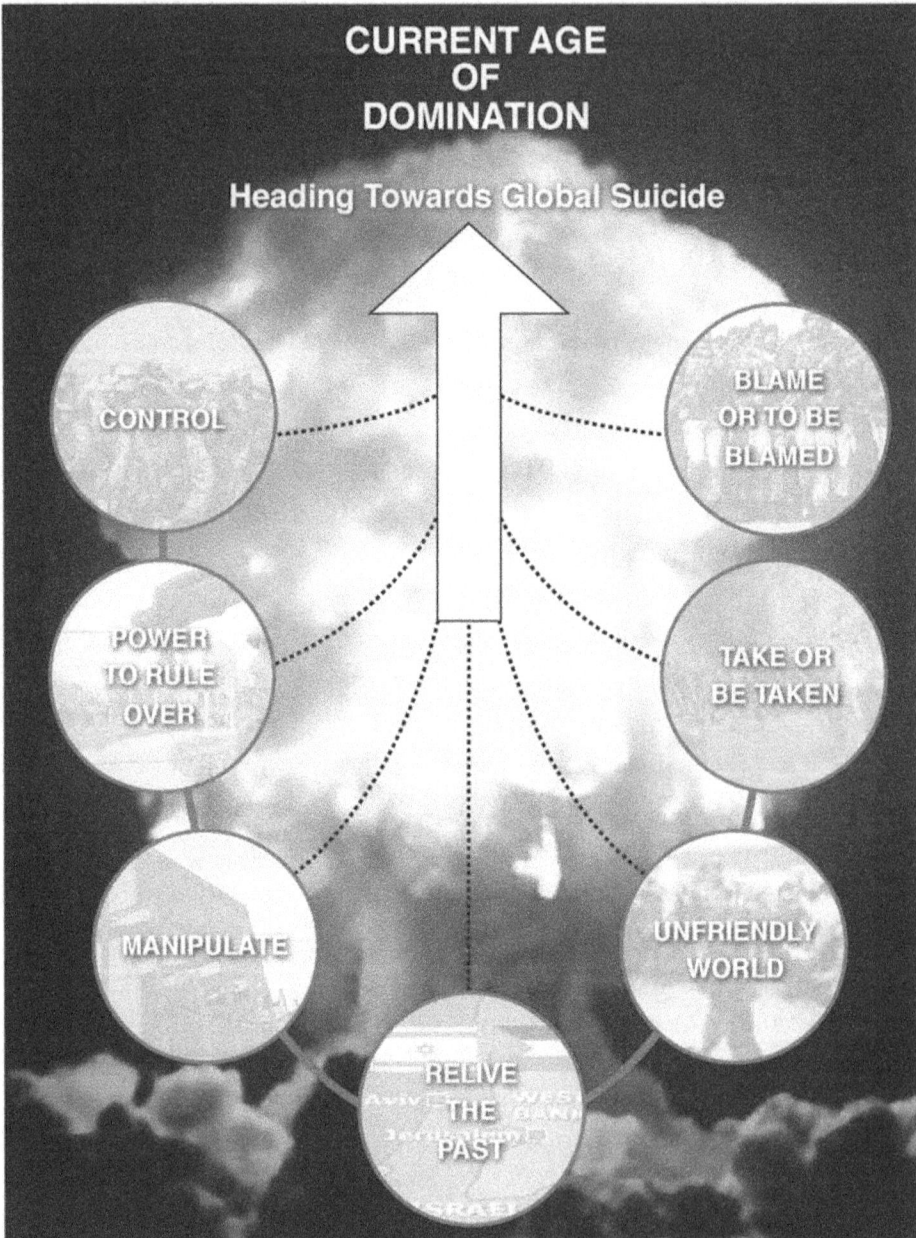

substantially and has added to terrorism.

Economically, the free enterprise system in the 20th century in democratic countries has passed through the agricultural revolution, industrial revolution and the high tech revolution, which has created wealth and prosperity. Gradually, the free enterprise system is taking hold in developing and communist countries. In spite of the creation of wealth, the gaps between the haves and have-nots increased and added fuel to recruitment of terrorists.

However, many underdeveloped countries are left behind and are still stricken by poverty, substandard living conditions and a lack of food, water and sanitary conditions. Meanwhile, industrialized countries spend trillions of dollars on military defense. This control is called "defense" because of insecurity and Domination. We talk about compassion and caring, but we spend more on control and Domination. How can we have compassion and caring when we like to control and dominate?

The second component of Domination is power to rule over others. If we do not have power over others, then someone will have power over us. If we do not impose our rules, if we do not stand up and claim our territories, someone else will and we will become their possession. We will come under their power.

Political, economic and religious leaders of the Global Family, paint this picture to justify their desire for power. Many of them relish ruling by instilling fear in other people, organizations and/or nations. They think this is the only way to ensure their security. They cannot think "outside the box" or think of other ways to create reality.

The third component of Domination is manipulation. The Webster Dictionary meaning of manipulate is, "to manage or control artfully or by shrewd use of influence, especially in an unfair or fraudulent way".

In the earlier years of history, Domination was enforced through physical power of individuals, soldiers and armies. Manipulation was applied through the skill of operating physical weapons such as swords, spears, arrows and other weapons.

In the modern age, manipulation of the members of the Global Family is mental, emotional and religious. Mental manipulation is generally called negotiation, using logic, reason, rationality, intellect and intelligence. Political campaigns, however, involve mental and emotional manipulation using mass media. In addition, organized religions manipulate members of the Global Family through the use of ignorance, greed, fear, doctrines and dogmas.

The fourth component of Domination is reliving the past in support of the negative ego. The Webster Dictionary meaning of ego is, "the self; the individual is aware of himself; conceit; in philosophy, variously conceived as an absolute spiritual substance on which experience is superimposed, the series of acts and mental states introspectively recognized; one's own personal interests almost to the exclusion of everything else; viewing everything in relation to oneself; self centered".

Metaphysically, the ego can be classified in two categories. One is the positive ego, which likes to grow mentally, emotionally and spiritually and is called "self". The other is called the negative ego, which dwells upon your personal interests almost to the exclusion of everything else.

The negative ego is self-centered and egocentric and cannot make new choices and decisions. It relies on established beliefs and attitudes of the past that come from the subconscious and unconscious mind. As discussed previously, the subconscious and unconscious minds like consistency. They enjoy reliving the past again and again in different forms.

Billions of dollars have been spent by Israel and Palestine to protect the holy land, yet there is no resolution for any of the issues. Using the same dollar amount that was spent in the war over the past fifty years, we could have created another holy land. It is all a matter of thinking "outside the box", creating new choices and decisions rather than reliving the past. We don't have to relive the past; we can create our own new reality.

The fifth component of Domination is living in an unfriendly world where the leaders of the Global Family have been supporting the negative ego on the pathway of Domination. They have created a mass psychology, and we have allowed them to do this in the belief that if you do not control others then others will control you; if you do not have power over others then someone will have power over us; that manipulation is the only way of living life; and creating the future depends on past experiences.

On this pathway of Domination we have now arrived at the 21st century and are living in a dangerous, scary and unfriendly world.

The sixth component of Domination is to take or be taken. Many people believe that they have to take things away from other people because if they do not, things will be taken from them. Their whole focus is on how much they are going to benefit from what is taken. Leaders on the pathway of Domination constantly think of what they can take and/or how they are being taken during all negotiations, treaties and agreements. They carry the constrictive consciousness of limited availability. They are not imaginative, innovative and inventive in creating more and therefore, being able to give.

Individually, a person occupying the position of Domination, while supporting and building the ego, generates constrictive emotions in all relationships. Usually these emotions are: fear, hurt, jealousy, envy, blame, revenge (violence), loneliness and despair. A dominant person generates fear in others and imprisons himself in the fear that he may lose control and the power to rule over others. He lives in a constant state of anxiety. His built up ego is motivated by false esteem through repression of thoughts and feelings and making choices out of fear.

A dominator generates hurt and pain in others by controlling and ruling over them. At the same time, he incubates hurt and pain within himself because of betrayal, abandonment, rejection and humiliation by others. A dominator feels as though there is rampant competition to control and have power over others by means of material wealth or by political, social, economic and religious position. He thrives on outside validation and generates the constricting emotions of jealousy and envy. He is jealous of what others have and covets what he does not have. He is envious of others because he feels that he is deprived of the happiness, joy, loving and caring which they have. His jealousy and envy boil to the point of rage and revenge, which then turns into violence. The built up ego of the dominator thrives on outside validation. At the same time, he feels empty and lonely.

A dominator indulges himself in having more and more control and power over others. In desperation, he becomes oppressive and repressive, making others feel helpless and hopeless as he imprisons himself in despair.

The seventh and final component in Domination is blame. In physical reality, a doctor prescribes an anesthetic to a patient suffering from severe pain. Similarly, a dominating person takes an anesthetic in the form of blaming others to numb their constricting emotions – fear, anxiety, hurt, jealousy, revenge, loneliness and despair - without taking any responsibility for creating the constricting emotions (see figure *"Anesthetic of Blame"*).

Therefore, a person is surrounded by the resonance of Domination searching for the pathway to develop and build the ego. The journey starts with control through manipulation to rule over and dominate others. This person develops and builds a repetitive pattern that eventually becomes a part of his subconscious mind. He creates beliefs and attitudes that Domination is the only way to live a successful life. Although physical forms change, the functions remain the same as he continues to relive the past. He conceives and perceives the world as an unfriendly place. He always looks to take from others and blame others for his reality.

The dominating person does not want to take the responsibility for reality. It is easier to blame than to take responsibility. Responsibility is hard work consisting of thinking, feeling, integrating, acting, imagining, making new choices and decisions, and developing the courage to take new directions into uncharted waters.

> *Collectively, after 9/11, our political, military, financial and religious leaders went through the motions of blaming others nationally and internationally. Even the United Nations started pointing fingers at each other in blame. They never recognized the possibility that we, the leaders and members of the Global Family, created this reality and we are responsible for it. Now is the time to take responsibility to change the mindset of fanatics, win the war on terrorism and avoid Global Suicide.*

Currently, self-esteem, which is the fulcrum in the hierarchy of needs, is based on Domination. The progression of the Global Family is based on

Anesthetic of Blame

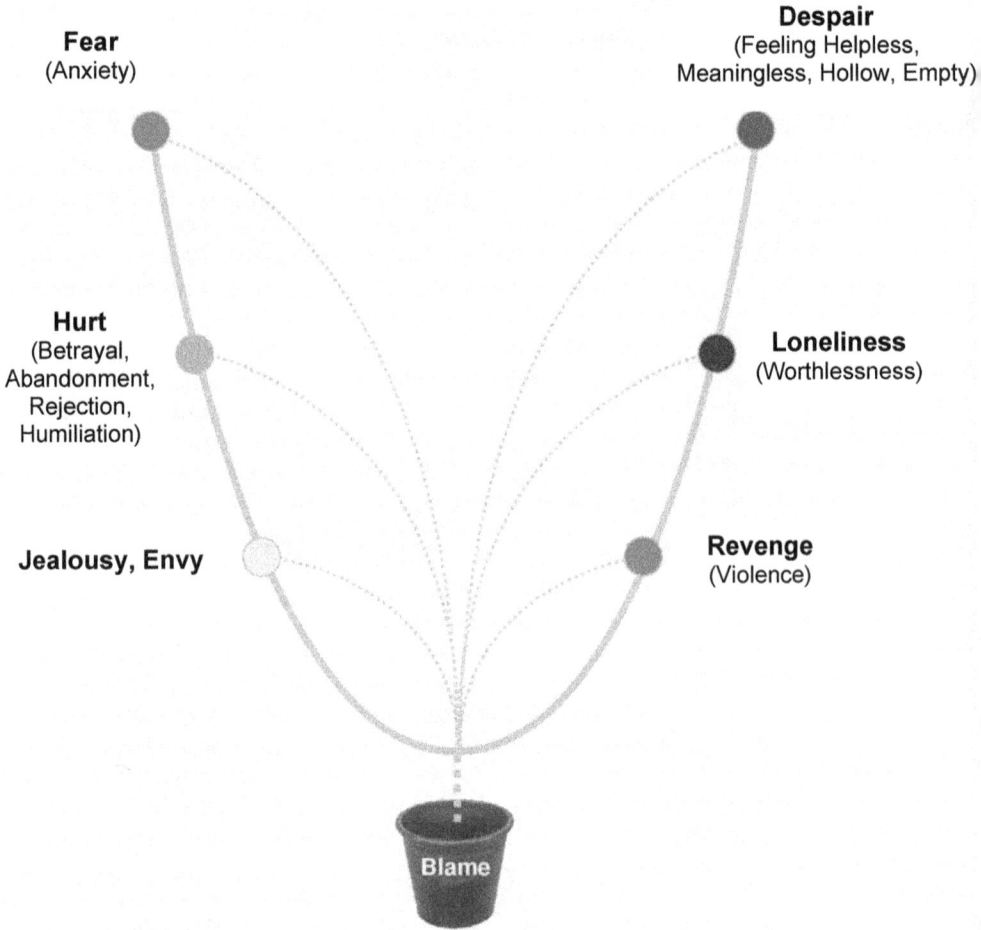

the principles of cooperation and co-creation among the members of the Global Family while healing the alliance of needs. However, the law of cooperation and co-creation has turned into comparison and competition. Leaders become competitive to maintain their positions and power by adopting the path of Domination. We, the members of the Global Family allow them to be on the path of Domination.

The path of Domination is a journey of the human ego. I am better than you. I am more than you. We are better than you. We are more than you. We can control, manipulate and rule over you. We don't need your cooperation, we can force our beliefs upon you. We are powerful. We are the chosen ones.

The Ways of Metaphysics are:

Individually:

I am the master of my destiny, and
not a victim of fate.

Collectively:

We, the members of the Global Family, are the masters of our destiny,
and not the victims of fate.

What is fate? According to the Webster Dictionary, fate is: "The power that is supposed to determine the inevitable outcome of events before they occur; hence inevitable necessity; destiny depending on superior cause, and uncontrollable; as according to the Stoics, every event is determined by fate; something inevitable, supposedly determined by this power; what happens or has happened to a person; lot; fortune."

What is destiny? According to the Webster Dictionary, destiny is: "State or condition appointed or predetermined; ultimate fate; lot; fortune; destination; a necessity or fixed order of things established, as by a divine decree, or by an indissoluble connection or causes and effects. That which determines events; said of either supernatural agency of necessity."

According to these definitions, fate and destiny are more or less synonymous.   Destiny contains fate, fortune, lot by chance, predetermined, inevitable events by necessity and unknown supernatural forces. Destiny is something that has or will happen because of fate, by necessity and uncontrollable unknown supernatural forces that are mysterious or mystical.

In general, destiny is something that has happened or will happen because of fate. Happening by fate means it is happening outside or beyond our control. Destiny is seen as our fate or lot in life rather than our chosen fortune. If it is seen as a fated fortune, it is considered to be predetermined or inevitable. It is defined as an unknown power that determines the course of events.

Metaphysically, destiny is our destination within the space-time dimension. It is the place we are going to, the reason that we are going there, and is also our motivation for heading there. Destiny is a point of consciousness: it has no beginning, no middle and no end. Destiny is neither static nor fixed. It is dynamic, and it is alive. It is living and breathing. It waxes and wanes, accelerates and decelerates. It is fluid and flexible, ever changing, ever shifting and ever growing. When we allow our destiny to be alive, it can be a major resource and reservoir of power and an astounding tool to broaden our potential.

Individually, I am the master of my own destiny and not a victim of fate.

How?

Destiny is a living matrix. Think of a standing wave of resonance emerging from the living matrix of fate, fortune, inevitable predetermination, and unknown energies and forces (see figure *"Emergence of Destiny As Resonance From the Four Components"*).

What is resonance? In physics, when two sound frequencies merge together, a new frequency emerges. As an example, if a musical instrument such as the sitar is tuned and a second sitar similarly tuned is played, the frequency of vibration from the second sitar being played will touch the first sitar causing it to play in a sympathetic vibration (see figure *"Physical Examples of Resonance"*).

141

Another example of resonance can be seen when two stones are dropped into a small lake a certain distance apart creating ripples, which at some point overlap and create an interference pattern (chaos). From there, a standing wave emerges.

An example of resonance that cannot be seen is when a man and woman are in a loving relationship, their thoughts and feelings overlap to create an interference pattern, which in turn creates the standing wave of resonance. This becomes a loving relationship (see figure "*Metaphysical Example of a Loving Man -Woman relationship*").

Fate

British Lord Bernard Shaw said that "by virtue of birth my father, mother, brother, sister, nephews, nieces, aunts and uncles and genetic/birth related siblings are fixed. Thank God you gave me the right to select my own friends, life partners and others."

So, there is a choice, there is will, there are desires, passions, challenges, dreams and visions. Fate can be changed. Fate is neither outside nor beyond our control. You are not a victim of fate. We are not victims of fate. It is not a huge mystery nor does it need to be. Fate can be designed, planned, programmed, processed and then manifested according to design by the power of will.

What is will? The Webster Dictionary defines will as: "power of self-direction; the power of conscious and deliberate action".

Metaphysically, will is the energy that has the ability to manifest reality. There are four kinds of will. The Hierarchy of Wills mirror the Hierarchy of Needs.

Emergence of Destiny as Resonance
From
The Four Components

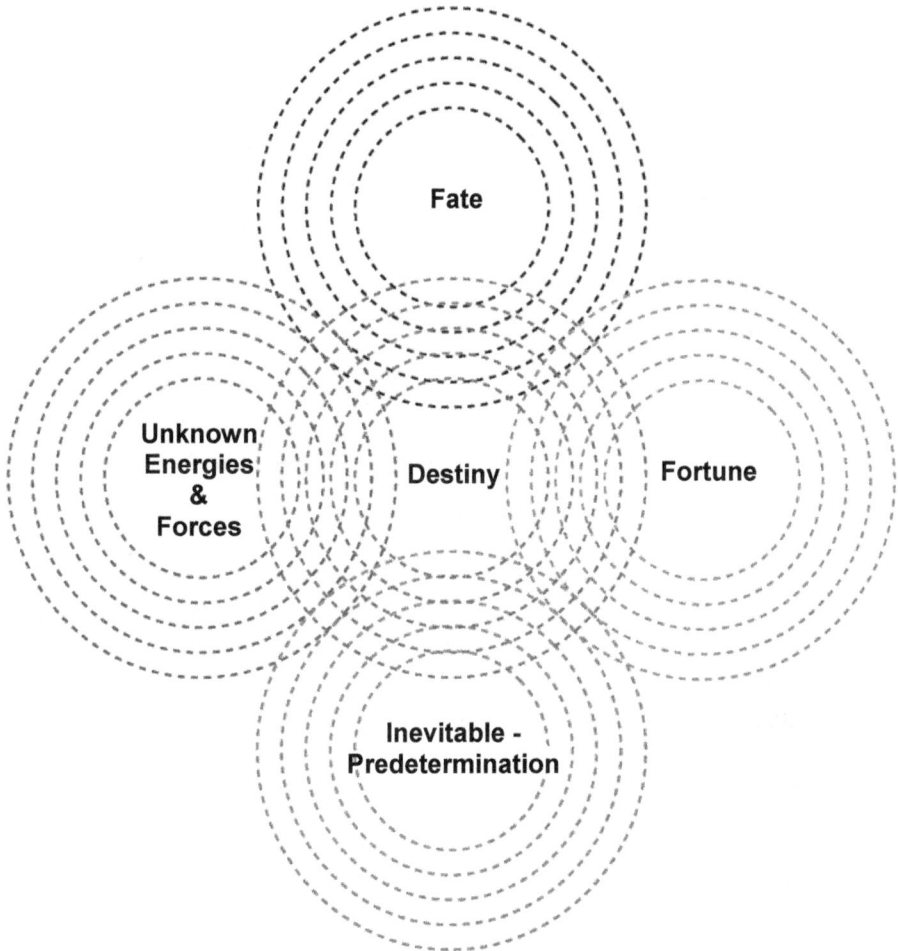

Physical Examples of Resonance

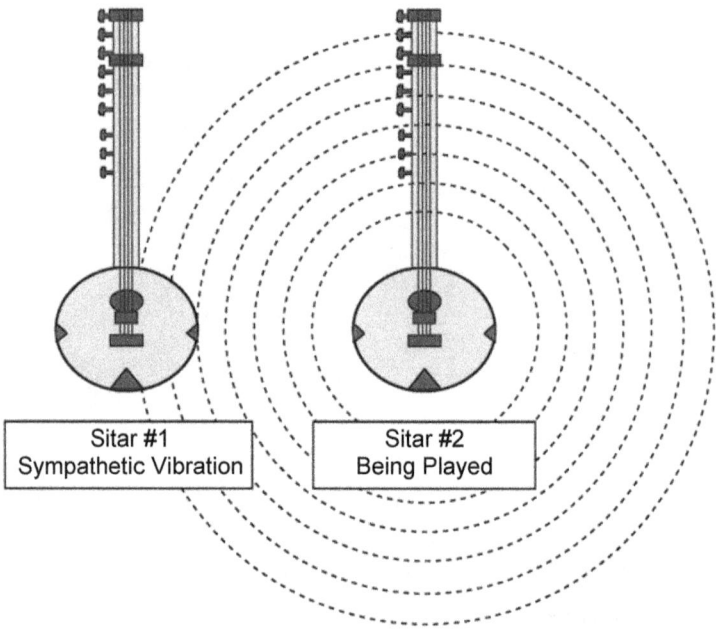

Sitar #1
Sympathetic Vibration

Sitar #2
Being Played

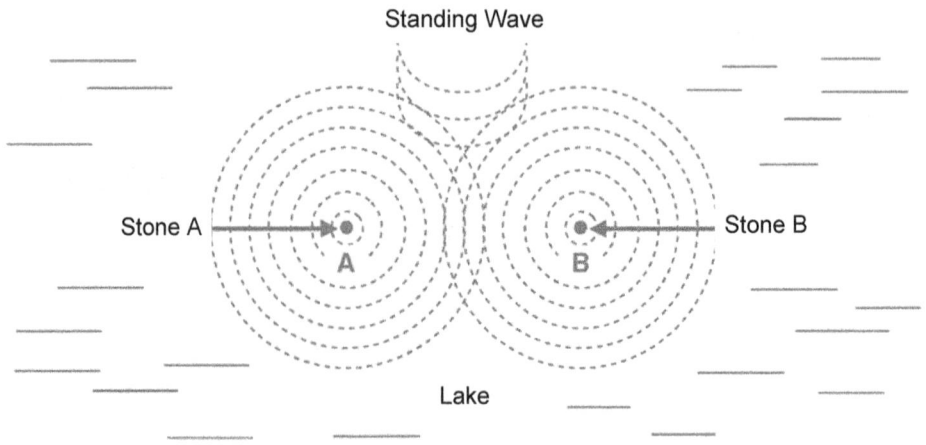

Standing Wave

Stone A

A

Stone B

B

Lake

Metaphysical Example
of
A Loving Man – Woman Relationship

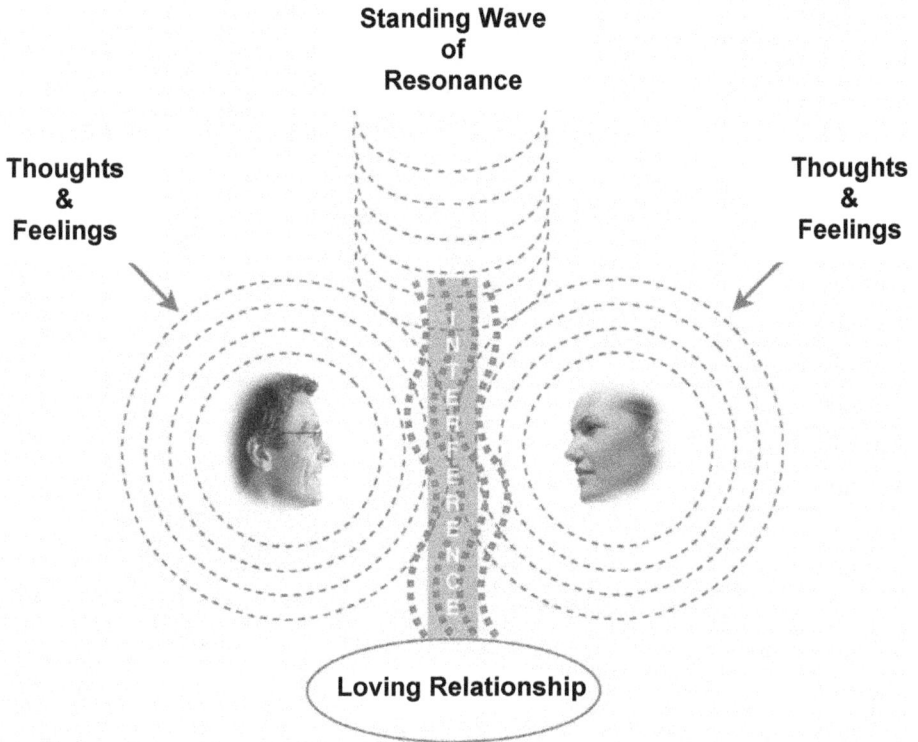

Standing Wave
of
Resonance

Thoughts
&
Feelings

Thoughts
&
Feelings

INTERFERENCE

Loving Relationship

The first kind of will is Instinctive or Automatic Will. Instinctive Will responds to the basic needs of survival, security and belonging. Instinctive Will has little or no power in making choices or decisions. Therefore, Instinctive Will uses choice to the first power, or Choice[1].

Geometrically, Choice[1] is called a point choice – ⬤

> *When you are driving a car, you encounter a potential accident. Your Instinctive Will takes over, and you physically take action to avoid the accident, therefore satisfying your need to survive.*

> *In the battlefield, the soldiers look for protection against the enemy, satisfying the need for physical security.*

> *In the civilized world, an employee looks for a permanent job satisfying the need for job security.*

> *When someone is asked "Who are you?" the person will instinctively reply "I am an engineer, doctor, lawyer or I am Christian, Jewish, Islamic or Hindu, Buddhist or Taoist." Satisfying the need to belong.*

The second kind of will is Wishing and Desiring Will. The will of wishing and desiring responds to the higher self-esteem and esoteric needs. The self-esteem need is creating, producing, and knowing, and the esoteric need is seeking beauty, balance, symmetry and asymmetry. Wishing and Desiring Will has well defined choices and decisions. Wishing and Desiring Will is the choice to the second power, or Choice[2].

Point Choices

Geometrically, it is called area choice –
Where the area choice is surrounded
and supported by the point choices.

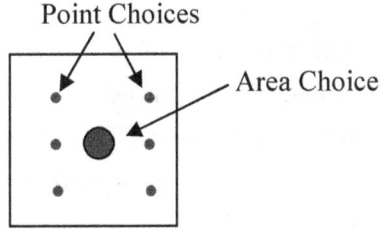

Area Choice

Let us practically apply the Wishing and Desiring Will to the guardians and leaders of the Global Family.

The subconscious mind of each guardian/leader of the Global Family says: "I have a wish and desire to become leader by taking the leadership position (fulfills the self-esteem need). I am capable of giving my services by taking the desired position. I will enjoy serving the people through this position. In this position, I use my inner wisdom and the ability to balance. This is my destiny (filling the esoteric need)."

They make a choice to acquire a position and to become the guardians and leaders of the Global Family.

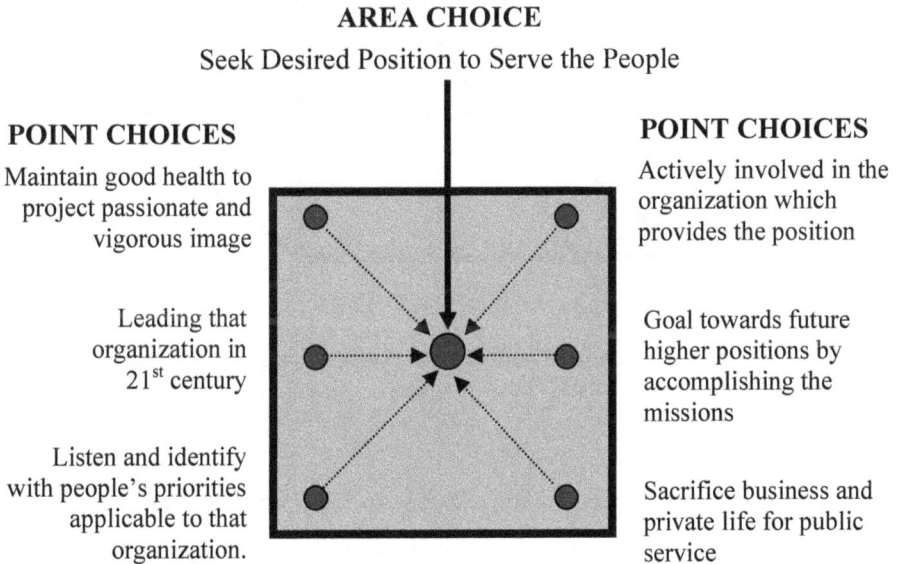

AREA CHOICE
Seek Desired Position to Serve the People

POINT CHOICES

Maintain good health to project passionate and vigorous image

Leading that organization in 21st century

Listen and identify with people's priorities applicable to that organization.

POINT CHOICES

Actively involved in the organization which provides the position

Goal towards future higher positions by accomplishing the missions

Sacrifice business and private life for public service

The third kind of will is Reflective Will. Reflective Will responds to personal preferences beyond basic and higher needs that come from dreams and visions. Decisions are vividly defined by dreams and visions and choices are made as fundamental choices from dreams and visions.

Geometrically, Reflective Will is called the fundamental choice or the volume choice, which is choice to the third power, or Choice[3]

Area Choice – Seeking the position of leadership to serve the people.

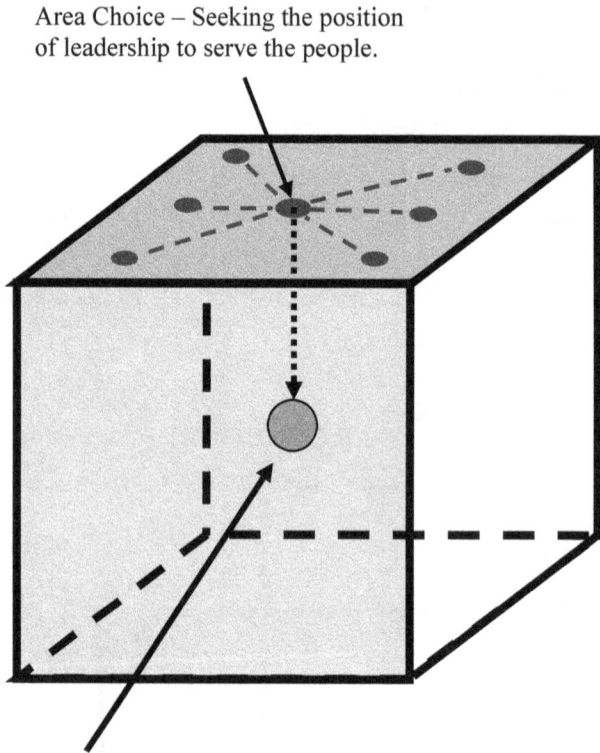

Fundamental Choice Coming from Preferences of Dreams and Visions (center of cube).

The fundamental choice is surrounded and supported by area choices, and area choices are in turn surrounded and supported by point choices.

Mahatma Gandhi had a dream. His dream was to liberate Indians from British rule. He heard the soul's call to adventure and pursued this dream of liberation through non-violence for more than forty years. India was finally liberated in 1947.

Dr. Martin Luther King also dreamed of liberating the African American minority from discrimination. He heard the soul's call to adventure and pursued his dream and vision. The Civil Rights Bill was passed in the 1960's.

Similarly, Nelson Mandela heard the soul's call to adventure to pursue the dream of removing apartheid in South Africa. In 1990, Nelson Mandela was released from 27 years of imprisonment and led the transition to the first multi-racial democracy in South Africa ending apartheid.

The fourth kind of will is True Will, which is synchronized with Divine Will, meaning that God's will and a person's will are one in the same.

So, destiny is something that has happened or will happen as a result of the network of wills, the matrix of fundamental choices that we have made, and the standing wave of resonance that emerges from fundamental choices. When we really understand destiny, we can see it differently, and it becomes something we can change. We can change fate by choice and resonance by the power of will.

Fortune
The general public (consensus reality) believes that fortune is more related to the meaning of your lot in life rather than to your relationship with abundance. The meaning of lot is "using an object in deciding a matter by chance or decision or choice arrived at by this means; regarded as verdict of chance." So your lot in life may be a burden, duty or

unpleasant obligation. What has been your lot in life can become your fortune, which signifies your relationship with abundance.

That relationship can be changed from negative to positive, and positive to even more positive. Metaphysically, abundance means dealing with your bounty with a sense of significance, dignity, freedom, presence, grace, responsibility and the sense that your abundance is enough.

Abundance is also connected to your sense of autonomy, from being free of pain, free of the past and being reliable and powerful. Of course, abundance also deals with giving, your capacity to give, to get, to give away and to give as an exalted act. It corresponds with your facility to actively and consciously co-create and your willingness to celebrate and be triumphant. So, good fortune is secured on a tripod of finding abundance, exalted giving and receiving graciously.

Abundance can be physical/material, mental, emotional and spiritual of which you can create as much as you want. This gives you a tremendous amount of power and energy so you can master your destiny rather than be a victim of your lot in life or a victim of chance.

Predetermined and Inevitable
Among consensus reality, destiny is seen as being predetermined or inevitable in accordance with karmic law. If this is true, what happens to your choices, your will, your dreams and visions of becoming something more, your desires and your passion?

Your so-called predetermined/inevitable destiny can be changed and made dynamic by accepting your passionate internal challenge to fulfill your desires to manifest your dreams and visions. Destiny can be altered when it is anchored by challenge, desire and passion moreso than when it is anchored by burden, duty and obligation.

By creating your own good fortune, you have an abundance of power and energy to accept challenges and manifest your desires using your passion while fulfilling your burdens, duties and obligations. Define yourself by challenging yourself, by your desires and passion, so you can determine and master your own destiny.

Unknown Power

Consensus reality thinks that destiny is an unknown power that determines the course of events. It carries the connotation that within the mystery of the unknown power, there is a debilitating quality. The unknown power that determines the course of events does not have to remain unknown. It can be known by your motivation to master it.

Enlightened motivation is much more than the motivation to fulfill your basic needs. Enlightened motivation reaches for the stages of self-esteem and esoteric needs, and drives one toward the attainment of true knowing and the fulfillment of their spiritual needs. It is the motivation to become multidimensional and multi-emotional, to seek the thrill and dominion in life, and become wise, free and eternal. Enlightened motivation is the unknown power, no longer unknown. It is your positive momentum. It is the perpetual motion of your love, will, intimacy and choice. The course of events can follow your motivation, your positive momentum, and can follow the maps you have made for yourself.

Destiny by Design and Direction

Destiny is a resonance of fate, fortune, inevitable and unknown power that directs the course of events. It is dynamic, ever changing and ever evolving. People often believe that either there is a destiny and we do not consciously create our own realities, or there is no destiny and we create it all. Yes, destiny is fate, which you consciously create by the power of your Reflective Will. It is the resonance that emerges from the network and the matrix of fundamental choices.

Yes, destiny is your fortune, but it is your good fortune that can be made consciously by finding your abundance and by consciously having gracious generosity, including the power of exalted giving and receiving of your abundance.

Yes, destiny is inevitable. You can create your destiny powerfully, positively and beautifully by anchoring yourself to your challenges, desires and passions.

Yes, destiny is a power that directs the course of events, which is the power of your motivation - your positive momentum and not an unknown power.

Destiny is the resonance of your willed fate, good fortune and "inevitables" determined by you and your power of motivation (see figure "*Destiny By Design And Direction*"). Destiny is a point of destination within the space-time dimension and a point of consciousness beyond the space-time dimension. Destiny is dynamic, alive, ever changing and ever evolving. It is not your enemy. It is your ally. Destiny is a tool that you can utilize to create a happy and successful reality. Destiny is a vibrant tool, which can be utilized for consciously directing the evolution of the Global Family towards Global Healing.

Evolution of the Human Race
Where are we heading? On this path of Domination, we will commit Global Suicide unless we consciously change the direction of the evolution of the Global Family by way of Metaphysics. It is important to understand the principles of evolution bringing us to this junction so that we can learn our lesson and consciously redirect evolution utilizing the power of destiny by design and direction (see figure "*Principles of Evolution*").

Destiny By Design and Direction

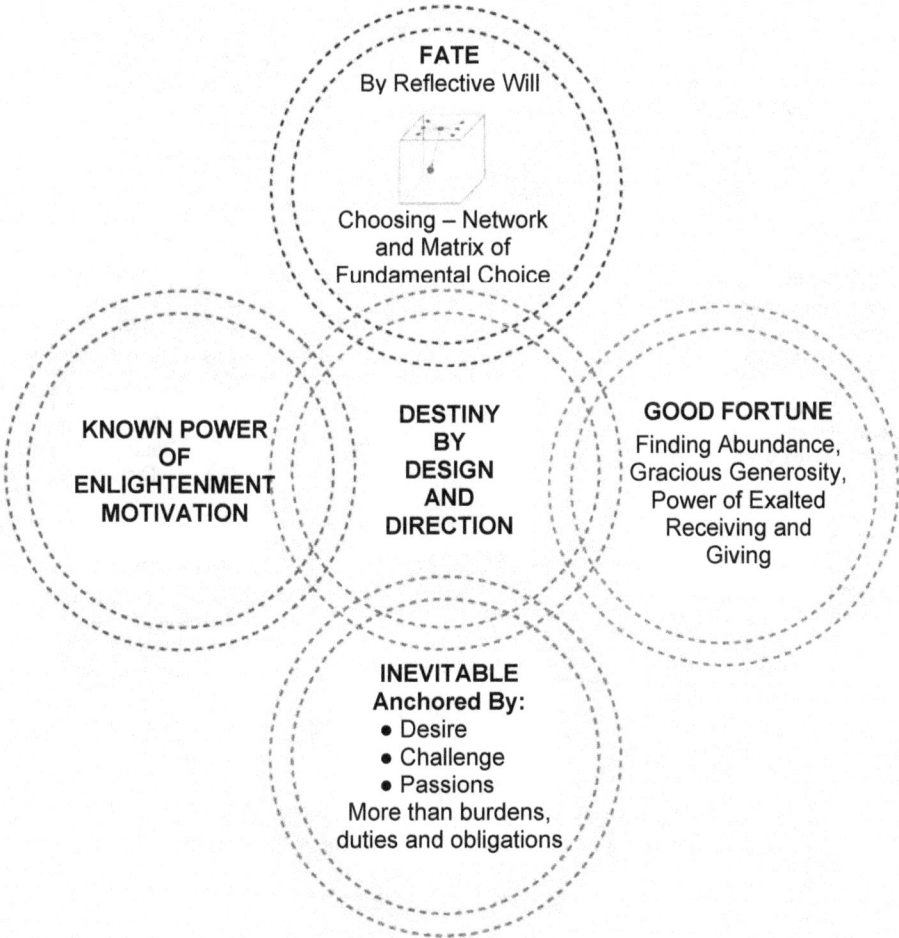

FATE
By Reflective Will

Choosing – Network
and Matrix of
Fundamental Choice

KNOWN POWER
OF
ENLIGHTENMENT
MOTIVATION

DESTINY
BY
DESIGN
AND
DIRECTION

GOOD FORTUNE
Finding Abundance,
Gracious Generosity,
Power of Exalted
Receiving and
Giving

INEVITABLE
Anchored By:
● Desire
● Challenge
● Passions
More than burdens,
duties and obligations

Principles of Evolution

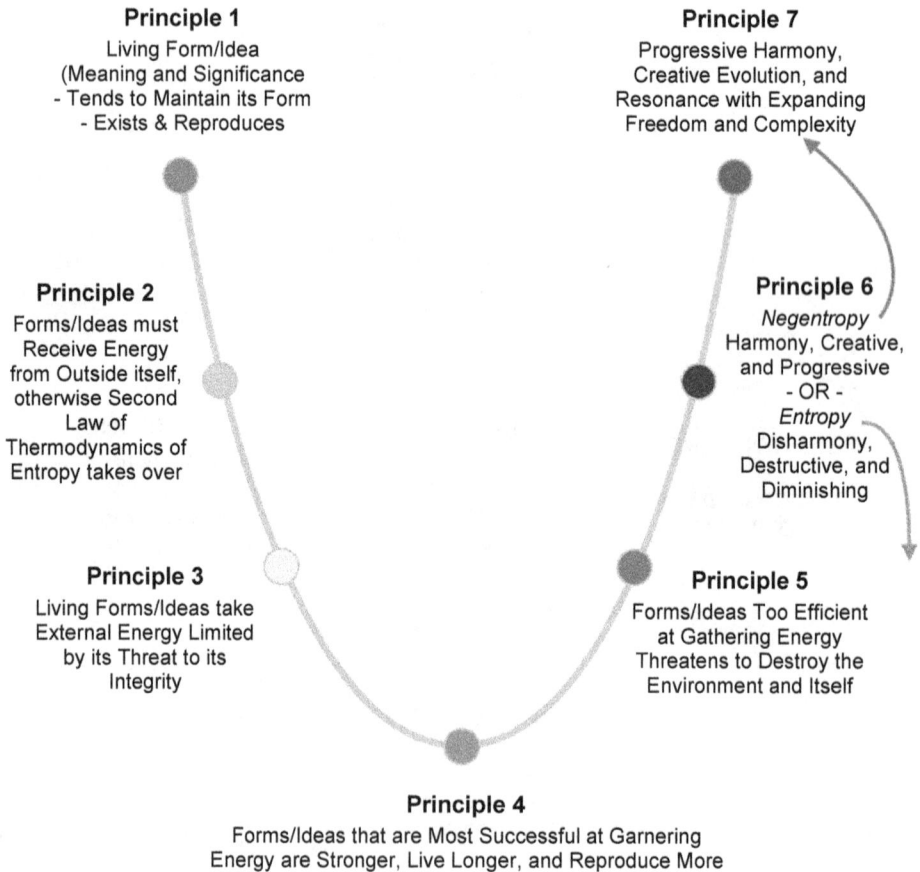

Principle 1

Living Form/Idea
(Meaning and Significance
- Tends to Maintain its Form
- Exists & Reproduces

Principle 7

Progressive Harmony,
Creative Evolution, and
Resonance with Expanding
Freedom and Complexity

Principle 2

Forms/Ideas must
Receive Energy
from Outside itself,
otherwise Second
Law of
Thermodynamics of
Entropy takes over

Principle 6

Negentropy
Harmony, Creative,
and Progressive
- OR -
Entropy
Disharmony,
Destructive, and
Diminishing

Principle 3

Living Forms/Ideas take
External Energy Limited
by its Threat to its
Integrity

Principle 5

Forms/Ideas Too Efficient
at Gathering Energy
Threatens to Destroy the
Environment and Itself

Principle 4

Forms/Ideas that are Most Successful at Garnering
Energy are Stronger, Live Longer, and Reproduce More

The first principle of evolution is that any form, be it physical or a thought or idea, becomes a living form and this form itself has meaning and significance. This living form has tendencies to exist, maintain itself, and reproduce.

> *Physically, plants, animals and humans are living forms on Earth. They have meaning and significance and they exist. They tend to maintain their forms themselves and then reproduce through built-in biological systems.*

> *Primitive man had a basic instinct for survival, influencing his thoughts and ideas. Survival was only possible by controlling his surrounding environment, including animals and other humans. This was the earliest form of Domination. The idea "to control" had meaning and significance for survival, existing, maintaining and reproducing its form among the human race.*

The second principle of evolution is that in order to exist, to be alive, to maintain its form and reproduce, the form or idea must receive energy from outside itself. Otherwise, the second law of the thermodynamics of entropy will take over. The law of entropy erodes, tears apart and causes the form or idea to decay. This is the aging process in human beings.

> *Physically, the human being is a very complex and intricate living and breathing form. We tend to stay alive, maintain our form and reproduce. To do so we need outside energy in the form of food, water, air, oxygen, nutrients and more.*

> *Although our ideas do not need food or oxygen, they do need the food of attention. The idea of Domination started with the basic need of survival and drew more attention in order to satisfy the second need of security. Therefore, the idea of Domination*

evolved further from control to the power to rule over others.

The third principle of evolution is that the form or idea will take as much external energy as possible, limited only by threats to its integrity of maintaining its form.

Human beings have complex integrity issues because they include physical form, state of mind, state of being and consciousness. The integrity of the human being also includes: the focus or purpose of life; identity of doing, feeling, thinking and expressing; image; and destiny. So, a human being will take as much energy as possible, limited only by that which threatens his/her physical being, conscious being and destiny. Models' intake of food is limited only by needing to stay thin and at the same time maintain that identity, image and destiny.

Ideas of Domination, control and the power to rule over others needs food of attention limited only by threats to its integrity. In the Second World War, Hitler focused on the idea of Domination of the Aryan race, to gain control and power over all of Europe and the world. He became overly ambitious, which destroyed his integrity, and he lost the war.

The fourth principle of evolution is that those forms or ideas that are more successful at garnering energy, grow stronger, live longer and reproduce more of themselves.

Human beings have the most evolved consciousness among the mineral, plant, animal and human kingdoms. They are the most successful in gathering energy, and therefore, they are stronger, live longer and reproduce more. In the 20th century, the human population increased substantially from 1.5 billion to 6 billion *people. Longevity has increased from an average of 55 years to 70 years. Humans are the strongest among all members of the planet.*

Similarly in the business world, products that have more marketability create more sales, last longer and are reproduced at a higher rate.

The ideas of democracy were established more than 225 years ago in the U.S. Democracy was very successful at the outset at garnering energy from the people and became stronger and stronger. In the 20th century, democracy entered into a competition with communism. Democracy gathered more energy by using the principles of freedom, liberty and justice for all. Democracy became stronger and stronger throughout the world, and communism lost ground as evidenced by the fall of the Berlin Wall and the disintegration of the USSR (Union of Soviet Socialist Republics).

The fifth principle of evolution is that when the previous four principles become too efficient at gathering energy from the environment, they can threaten to destroy the environment, and in turn, destroy themselves.

In the 20th century, the human race has made substantial progress in gathering energy from the environment thanks to the advances of science and technology. Although these advances have helped our economy grow, many of them have also seriously threatened our environment. We have become so efficient at outputting greenhouse gasses and destroying forests and have upset the balance in the cycle of carbon dioxide and oxygen. The world is suffering from air and water pollution and the survival of all living things is being threatened.

157

The human race has become tremendously efficient in reproducing. Every twelve years we produce one billion more people. This rate of reproduction is a population explosion, which actually threatens the human race itself.

During the last one hundred years, Domination has become "too efficient" through the use of the previous four principles of evolution by gathering and shifting the energy of attention. This has created the mass psychology that Domination is the only way of bringing resolution to the conflicts of the Global Family. Although the forms of Domination are constantly being refined with increased complexity, the function of Domination remains the same.

The sixth principle of evolution is that when the fifth principle becomes too efficient, evolution can move in either of two directions. It can move to disharmony and entropy in a downward spiral of destruction, or it can move toward harmony and negentropy in an upward spiral of creation. The first direction can be called diminishing and the second can be called progressive.

If the human race remains too efficient in drawing the energy from it's environment by burning oil, cutting down forests, polluting the air and water; depleting the fertility of land; adulterating the food with hormones; and not controlling the population explosion, then the well being of the human race will steadily diminish. This is the path of disharmony, entropy and destruction.

If the human race uses the ways of Metaphysics, we can consciously direct evolution toward the path of harmony, negentropy and creation by utilizing destiny by design. This is progressive evolution leading us toward Global Healing.

The seventh principle of evolution is progress. The evolution of progress can be assured by creating resonance by expanding freedom and expanding complexity under unifying principles. Generally, there are three types of resonance: random chance (accident), necessity, and random selection (lottery). These types are caused by nature. We can also create resonance by conscious choice. This conscious choice is utilizing destiny by design and direction for the progress of evolution.

On the path of Domination, the cycle of living in two periods, preparation for war and war itself, has become overly efficient with the advancement of science and technology. This brought the Global Family from the fifth to the sixth principle of evolution, where we are currently situated. As it stands now, we are coming even closer to the evolution of deterioration through entropy instead of the evolution of progress through negentropy. If we choose the evolution of progress through harmony and creation, the dawning of the new Age of Dominion would then be at hand.

It is also generally believed that the present emerges from the past leading towards the unknown or projected future. But intrinsically, the present emerges from the future in the backdrop of the past. The future is unknown so people generally look to the past to understand the emerging present. Using a lantern as a metaphor, if you leave your key under the lantern, and look for the key around the lantern where there is light (known past), but never look under the lantern where there is no light (unknown future), you will not find it. Similarly we look to the past to understand the present rather than relating the present to the future.

There is a well-known song by Doris Day, "Que sera, sera; whatever will be, will be. The future is not yours to see. Que sera, sera." Many people believe in this saying, and they just wait until the future shows up as the present and then deal with it. They also live in the present, moment to moment, without a sense of the future and without taking any responsibility for the future.

Successful people look to their dreams to create what they want to manifest in the future. Dreaming is natural to the human being and is part of human life. Conscious dreaming starts with imagination, and repeating patterns in our imagination becomes visualization. When visualization penetrates the subconscious and unconscious mind, it becomes part of dreaming. Dreams can be daydreams, lucid dreams or night dreams. It is said that anything that becomes physical reality first has to be perceived as an image and then transformed to reality. All successful people have dreams and visions. Their enlightened motivation made them successful in manifesting those dreams and visions. Throughout the process of bringing dreams to reality, the successful people remain anchored with the passionate desire to rise to challenges. Dr. Martin Luther King was well known for his phrase "I have a dream" which he kept in focus. Dreaming and visioning for the brighter and luminous future of the Global Family is the dawning of the new Age of Dominion.

Why is the brighter and luminous future so important? All successful people look into the future, dream of the future, focus on the future and passionately desire realizing their dreams in the future. They live and breathe the way of Metaphysics:

The future creates the present in the backdrop of the past
(downward causation), rather than believing the past creates
the present moving toward the future (upward causation).

They live in the present with the presence of the future, and
their dreams and visions create their success.

160

That is their secret.

We, the members of the Global Family, can use the secrets of successful people to dream and envision the dawning of a new Age of Dominion. We can rise to the challenge and win the war on terrorism while establishing Global Healing. Why can't the leaders and the guardians of the Global Family at the United Nations dream, envision and create a mission statement for the new age? This is our Reflective Will coming out of our preferences of dreams and visions creating the network and living matrix of fundamental choices (see figure *"Fate of Global Family Determined By Reflective Will"*). Ours is not 'mission impossible'. It is possible if we are focused by our passionate desire to accomplish it, rising above the challenges, and are driven by the fervent motivation to satisfy spiritual needs. When spirituality guides science and technology, then we will create an abundance of the energy and forces of good fortune. With good fortune we will have enough abundance to share graciously with others. This in turn will reduce the gaps between the haves and have-nots, between the hopeful and hopeless, those being helped and the helpless and the rational thinkers and fanatics. We can create destiny by design and direction, co-creatively working together.

In the way of Metaphysics: **The future creates the present in the backdrop of the past (downward causation).** It is the future, not the past that motivates growth and change. When someone has hope for the future, they feel it and sense it beyond fantasy. Changes happen and growth begins. The future is the motivator for all change and growth.

It is the future that determines the "realness", what is too much, too little or just right. The future can make the present more real, and it can make the past less real. The future holds that power. It is the future and the will to live that is the source of healing. It is the sense of future that allows medicine to heal patients.

Fate of Global Family Determined by Reflective Will

Area Choice of the U.N.
Member Nations Developing
Hope of Dawning the New
Age of Dominion

Point Choices Consciously
Create Global Healing by
Reducing Gaps

We are one Global
Family, all colors, all
races, one world united.
Through diversity we
recognize our unity

Fundamental
Choice/Mission
Statement of the
United Nations
Leading the Global
Family

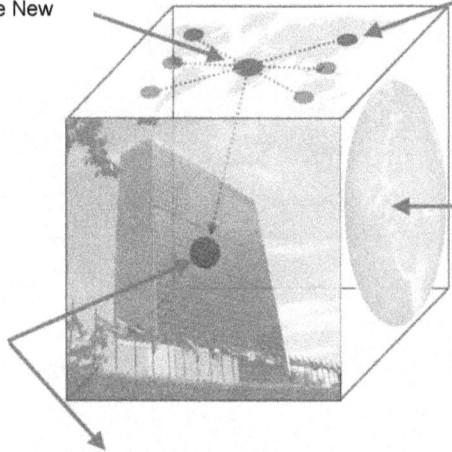

Dream State of Global Family
Dawning of the New Age of Dominion

The dawning of the new Age of Dominion is
where we can consciously co-create our own reality
without fighting for control over each other;

Where we will have power of collaboration
and the ability to help create global healing;

Where our spirituality will lead science and technology so they can
serve the global family rather than the be victims of weapons of mass
destruction;

Where the global family will be loving and have the ability to create
a brighter, luminous future rather than wallowing in past mistakes;

Where the world will be a friendly place
where people trust and help each other to build new creations
rather than an unfriendly place full of fear and distrust;

Where we will have the ability to create abundance
and to give and share with others, rather than to take and be taken;

Where we will love and care for each other,
rather than blame or find ourselves being blamed by others.

162

THE WAYS OF METAPHYSICS: PORTALS TO THE FUTURE

It is the future that gives value to life, which is beyond meaning and significance. In this space-time dimension and this world, so many things have meaning and significance, but if they do not change you, then they are of no value to you. So 'values' which change you, go beyond the space-time dimension. The future gives value to your life, which allows you to grow and change.

It is the future that empowers your choice and will. It is the future that takes you from the Wishing and Desiring Will, coming out of self-esteem and esoteric needs, to the Reflective Will that comes out of dreams and visions. It is the future that reveals who you truly are, your True Will.

The future is the resource for changing your current reality to a more positive, brighter, luminous reality.

The ways of Metaphysics are:

Individually:

> *"I create my own reality, and I am responsible for what I am.*
> *I am the master of my destiny, and not a victim of fate."*

Collectively:

> *"We, the members of the Global Family, create our own reality, and*
> *we are responsible for what we are.*
> *We, the members of the Global Family, are the masters of our destiny,*
> *and not victims of fate."*

Now is the time to open the portals to the future and allow the energies and the forces of the future to flow through our lives and extinguish the stale, stagnant, and polluted energies and forces of the past. We can live in the present with the presence of a brighter, luminous future in the new

Age of Dominion while releasing the burden of the past Age of Domination. The next two books will further open these portals to the future by discussing how to consciously create Global Healing by *Awakening Spirituality* and envisaging *New Vistas of Hope* as we work toward dawning a new Age of Dominion.

ABOUT THE AUTHOR

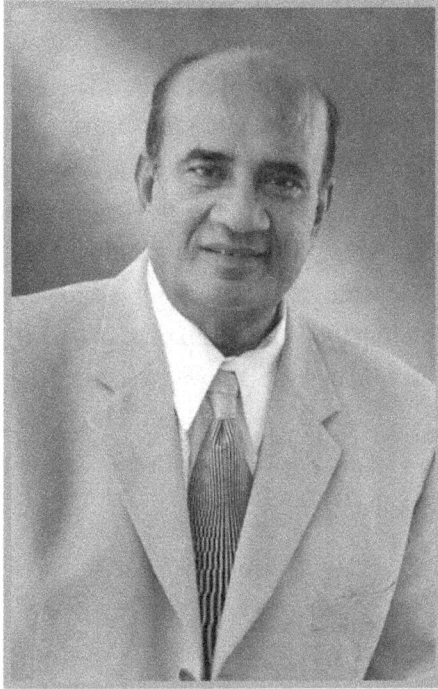

Vipin Mehta, P.E., M.A.P.A. was born in India and raised in Mumbai during the Independence Movement inspired through Mahatma Gandhi's principles of non-violence. Shortly after migrating to the United States in 1969 with only a few dollars to his name, Vipin became a licensed Professional Engineer and established *MEHTA Engineering*, which has since evolved into a 30-year engineering and construction management firm for roads, bridges, airports, and other infrastructure related projects. After arriving to the U.S., Vipin also received a Masters in Public Affairs from Northern Illinois University and has since played a very active role in local, state and national politics and has been addressed as the Metaphysical and Spiritual Counselor to many politicians – both Democrat and Republican.

Vipin has pursued Metaphysical and Spiritual learning by Spiritual Masters and Mystics from all over the world. His interest in Metaphysics began in 1947, where he first learned from Mahatma Gandhi's teachings. Other Spiritual Masters include the Indian mystics J. Krishnamurti, Rabindranath Tagore (Nobel Prize winner in 1912) and Rajneesh/Osho along with western spiritualists Edgar Cayce, Ruth Montgomery, and other modern mystics. Vipin has studied many Metaphysical and Spiritual scriptures including Hinduism, Buddhism, Taoism, Jainism, Sikhism, Zen, Christianity, Judaism, Islam, Sufi and others through which he taught "Religion of Man" courses at local Colleges and gave lectures on Metaphysics across the U.S. and India.

Vipin now lives in Orlando, Florida with his wife Hansa and has two children Ravé and Radha.